EMS Respiratory Emergency Management

DeMYSTiFieD

Peter A. DiPrima, Jr.

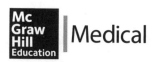

Medical

New York   Chicago   San Francisco   Athens   London   Madrid
Mexico City   Milan   New Delhi   Singapore   Sydney   Toronto

EMS Respiratory Emergency Management Demystified

Copyright © 2014 by McGraw-Hill Education, Inc. All rights reserved. Printed in the United States of America. Except as permitted under the United States Copyright Act of 1976, no part of this publication may be reproduced or distributed in any form or by any means, or stored in a data base or retrieval system, without the prior written permission of the publisher.

1 2 3 4 5 6 7 8 9 0   DOC/DOC   18 17 16 15 14 13

ISBN 9780071820837
MHID 0071820833

This book was set in Berling by Cenveo® Publisher Services.
The editors were Andrew Moyer and Christina M. Thomas.
The production supervisor was Richard Ruzycka.
Project management was provided by Sheena Uprety, Cenveo Publisher Services.
RR Donnelley was the printer and binder.

Notice

Medicine is an ever-changing science. As new research and clinical experience broaden our knowledge, changes in treatment and drug therapy are required. The authors and the publisher of this work have checked with sources believed to be reliable in their efforts to provide information that is complete and generally in accord with the standard accepted at the time of publication. However, in view of the possibility of human error or changes in medical sciences, neither the editors nor the publisher nor any other party who has been involved in the preparation or publication of this work warrants that the information contained herein is in every respect accurate or complete, and they disclaim all responsibility for any errors or omissions or for the results obtained from use of the information contained in this work. Readers are encouraged to confirm the information contained herein with other sources. For example and in particular, readers are advised to check the product information sheet included in the package of each drug they plan to administer to be certain that the information contained in this work is accurate and that changes have not been made in the recommended dose or in the contraindications for administration. This recommendation is of particular importance in connection with new or infrequently used drugs.

Library of Congress Cataloging-in-Publication Data

DiPrima, Peter A., Jr.
    Airway and respiratory emergency management demystified/Peter A. DiPrima Jr.
       p. ; cm.
    Includes bibliographical references and index.
    ISBN-13: 978-0-07-182083-7 (pbk.)
    ISBN-10: 0-07-182083-3 (pbk.)
    I. Title.
    [DNLM: 1. Airway Obstruction—therapy. 2. Emergencies. WF 145]
    RM161
    615.8′36—dc23
                                 2013014106

McGraw-Hill Education books are available at special quantity discounts to use as premiums and sales promotions, or for use in corporate training programs. To contact a representative please e-mail us at bulksales@mcgraw-hill.com.

To my father, who at the time of me writing this book was suffering from Small Cell Lung Cancer, thank you for all you have done. I am the person I am today because of you.

1948-2013, RIP! I love you Dad!

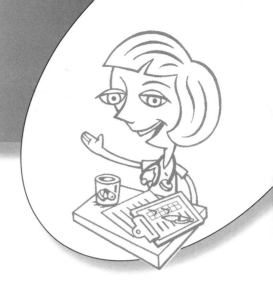

Contents

Preface   ix
Acknowledgment   x

CHAPTER 1   **Anatomy and Physiology of the Respiratory System**   1
The Respiratory System   2

CHAPTER 2   **Acid-Base Balance, Blood Gas Analysis**   33
Scenario   34
Introduction   34
Oxyhemoglobin Dissociation Curve   52

CHAPTER 3   **Pathophysiology of Apnea and Hypoxia**   61
What is Hypoxia   62

CHAPTER 4   **Pulse Oximetry and Capnography; What's the difference?**   71
Introduction   72
Principles of Pulse Oximetry   83

CHAPTER 5   **Oxygen Delivery Devices and Bag-Valve-Mask Ventilation**   93
Introduction   94

CHAPTER 6   **Respiratory Pharmacology**   109
Scenario   110
Introduction   111
Anatomy of the Autonomic Nervous System   112

CHAPTER 7	**Respiratory Emergencies**	**141**
	Scenario	142
	Respiratory Patterns	142
	Lung Sounds	142
	Asthma	142
	Chronic Obstructive Pulmonary Disease	144
	Chronic Bronchitis	144
	Emphysema	145
	Pulmonary Edema	147
	Pneumonia	150
	Respiratory Failure	155
CHAPTER 8	**Rapid Sequence Intubation**	**165**
	Introduction	166
	Rapid Sequence Induction versus Rapid Sequence Intubation	166
	Pharmacology: Sedative Agents for Rapid Sequence Intubation	175
	Patients and Findings	189
	Conclusions	190
	Summary	190
CHAPTER 9	**Endotracheal Intubation**	**193**
	Scenario	194
	Introduction	194
	Indications for endotracheal intubation	195
	Specific Criteria for Intubation	195
	Summary	214
CHAPTER 10	**Airway Devices for Difficult Airway Management, Supraglottic Airway Devices**	**217**
	Scenario	218
	Introduction	218
	Laryngeal Mask Airway	219
CHAPTER 11	**Special Clinical Considerations for the "Difficult Airway"**	**233**
	Epidemiology	234
	Airway Management of the Adult Trauma Patient	256
	Emergency Airway Evaluation of the Burn Patient	262
	Airway Management in Pregnancy	265
	Introduction	265

Anatomic and Physiological Changes
during Pregnancy   266
Morbid Obesity in Pregnancy and Airway   268
Difficult Airway Management in Bariatric Patients   268
Introduction   269
Pulmonary Physiology   269
Managing the Difficult Airway in Geriatric
Patients   272
Introduction   272
Cricothyroidotomy Surgical Airway   273
Introduction   274

CHAPTER 12   **Continuous Positive Airway Pressure (CPAP)**   **283**
Scenario   284
Introduction   284
Pathophysiology of Pulmonary Edema   285

Index   295

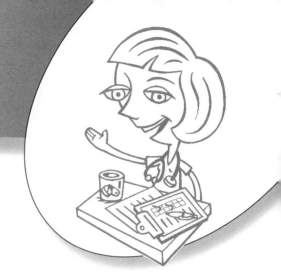

Preface

Guided by the patient's presenting complaint, this book emphasizes a methodical approach to patient evaluation, treatment, and problem solving during a respiratory emergency or complicated airway management. Unlike other books that elaborate on known diagnoses, this extraordinary book approaches clinical problems as clinicians approach patients–without full knowledge of the final diagnosis. This text effectively reveals how to address patients with respiratory conditions, ask the right questions, perform directed physical examination, and accurately perform lifesaving procedures.

EMS Respiratory Emergency Management Demystified is an important resource to emergency medical technician (EMT) and paramedic students, and will serve as an invaluable resource for practicing EMTs and paramedics. I hope you enjoy my book.

PAD

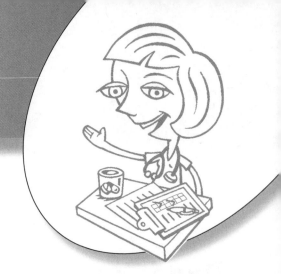

Acknowledgment

Apart from the efforts of myself, the success of any book depends largely on the encouragement and guidelines of many others. I take this opportunity to express my gratitude to the people who have been instrumental in providing guidance and support.

I am grateful for their constant support and help.

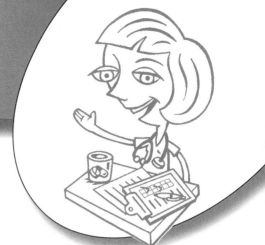

chapter 1

Anatomy and Physiology of the Respiratory System

LEARNING OBJECTIVES

At the end of this chapter, you will be able to:

1. Describe the primary functions of the respiratory system.

2. Explain how respiratory surfaces are protected from pathogens, debris, and other hazards.

3. Describe the anatomy of the upper airway and describe their functions.

4. Describe the anatomy of the lower anatomy and describe the structure and function of the lungs.

5. Discuss the function of the lymphatic system and how it relates to the lungs.

6. State the structures and functions of the pulmonary vascular system.

7. Describe gross lung anatomy including lobes, segments, and fissures.

8. State the important anatomic features of the thorax including pertinent bones, cartilage, and muscles.

⑨ List and describe the primary and accessory muscles of inhalation and exhalation.

⑩ Identify and discuss the brain centers involved with the control of ventilation.

⑪ Explain the factors that control ventilatory drive and respiratory rate.

⑫ Describe the physical principles governing the movement of gases conducted through the lung and into the blood stream.

⑬ Describe the two transport systems that the blood has for oxygen and carbon dioxide.

⑭ List and give normal volumes and capacities for the typical lung.

KEY TERMS

Adventitia
Bronchi
Bronchioles
Cartilage
External respiration
Hilus
Internal respiration
Laryngopharynx
Laryngospasm
Mucous membrane

Nasopharynx
Oropharynx
Pharyngeal wall
Pleura
Pleural cavity
Pleural fluid
Primary bronchi
Pulmonary ventilation
Type I alveolar cell
Type II alveolar cell

The Respiratory System

The primary function of the respiratory system is to supply the blood with oxygen. The respiratory system does this through breathing. When we breathe, we inhale oxygen and exhale carbon dioxide. This exchange of gases is the respiratory system's means of getting oxygen to the blood.

Why do cells need a continuous supply of oxygen?

Cells need a continuous supply of oxygen for the metabolic reactions that release energy from nutrient molecules and produce adenosine triphosphate (ATP). Oxygen is the final electron acceptor in oxidative phosphorylation.

Why must the body rid itself of carbon dioxide?

Carbon dioxide is produced during metabolism and is intimately involved in the formation of hydrogen ions in the body fluids. This produces acidity and is therefore toxic. It must be removed from the body quickly and efficiently.

What two systems work together to accomplish these tasks?

The cardiovascular and respiratory systems work together to accomplish these tasks.

What is the primary function of the respiratory system?

The essential function of the respiratory system is to provide for the exchange of gases between the atmosphere and the lungs, and between the lungs and the blood flowing through them.

There are at least four other less vital functions performed by the respiratory system.

1. Contains receptors for the sense of smell
2. Filters, warms, and moistens inspired air
3. Produces sound
4. Helps eliminate wastes other than carbon dioxide

The exchange of gases between the atmosphere, the blood, and the body cells is called respiration.

- Pulmonary ventilation: Pulmonary ventilation is breathing; the inspiration and expiration of air between the atmosphere and the lungs.
- External respiration: External respiration is the exchange of gases between the lungs and the blood.
- Internal respiration: Internal respiration is the exchange of gases between the blood and the body cells.

Compare the upper respiratory system with the lower respiratory system.

The respiratory system may be divided in several ways: upper versus lower, or conducting versus respiratory.

- The upper respiratory system refers to the nose, pharynx, and associated structures.
- The lower respiratory system refers to the larynx, trachea, bronchi, and lungs.

Compare the conducting portion of the respiratory system with the portions of the respiratory system.

- The conducting portion of the respiratory system consists of a system of interconnected cavities and tubes whose role is in actual gas exchange with the atmosphere (from the nose through the bronchi).
- The respiratory portion of the system consists of those portions where gas exchange with the blood actually occurs: from the respiratory bronchioles to the alveoli.

Anatomy and Physiology of the Respiratory System Organs

Nose (Anterior)

External nose: The external nose consists of a bone and cartilage framework covered with muscle and skin and lined with a mucous membrane. On its underside are the external nares (nostrils); see Figure 1-1a.

Internal nose: The internal nose is a large cavity in the skull that is inferior to the floor of the cranium and superior to the mouth. Anteriorly it merges with the external nose while posteriorly it opens into the pharynx via the internal nares. It receives the nasolacrimal ducts and the ducts of the paranasal sinuses (see Figure 1-1a).

Nasal cavity: The inside of the external and internal nose is the nasal cavity, divided into right and left sides by a vertical partition called the nasal septum. The anterior portion of the nasal cavity, just inside the nostrils, is an area called the vestibule. It is surrounded by cartilage and covered by skin (see Figure 1-1a).

Nasal conchae: From each of the lateral walls of the nasal cavity are three shelves or projections called superior, middle, and inferior nasal conchae, which reach medially almost to the nasal septum. Each concha is curved downward in a small spiral that subdivides the right and left nasal cavities into groove-like passageways (see Figure 1-1a).

Physiology: The interior structures of the nose are specialized for three functions.

1. Incoming air is filtered, moistened, and warmed: When air enters the nostrils, it passes first through the vestibule where large dust particles are filtered out by the coarse guard hairs located there. As the air moves past the conchae, it is swirled and exposed to the large surface area of the mucous membrane where smaller dust particles and other matter in the air become stuck. Cilia, a hair-like structure located in the mucous membrane, sweep the mucous and accumulated particles to the pharynx where they

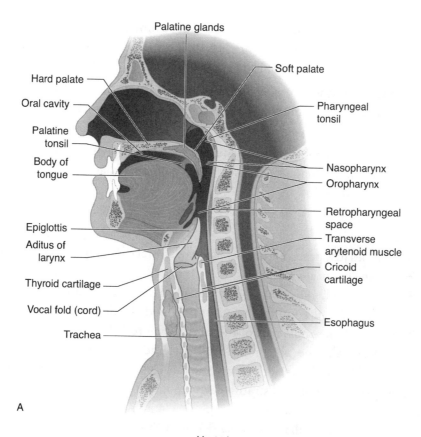

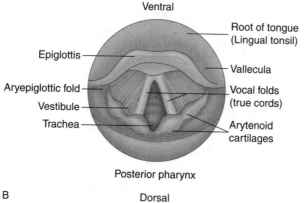

Figure 1-1 • Upper airway human anatomy.
(A) Reproduced with permission from Tintinalli JE, Stapczynski JS, Cline DM, Ma OJ, Cydulka RK, Meckler GD, eds. *Tintinalli's Emergency Medicine: A Comprehensive Study Guide.* 7th ed. 2001. New York: Copyright © McGraw-Hill Education. All rights reserved.
(B) Reproduced with permission from Reichman EF, Simon RR. *Emergency Medicine Procedures.* New York: Copyright © McGraw-Hill Education. All rights reserved.

can be swallowed. In addition, the mucous membrane is moist and has an extensive capillary network. This causes the air to be moistened and warmed as it passes through the nasal cavity.

2. Olfactory epithelium: The olfactory epithelium, located in the roof of the nasal cavity in the mucous membrane of the superior nasal conchae and along the septum, provides the sense of smell.

3. Resonating chambers: The chambers of the nasal cavity, along with those forming the paranasal air sinuses, form resonating chambers used to modify speech sounds.

Pharynx

Location: It lies just posterior to the nasal cavity, oral cavity, and larynx, and just anterior to the cervical vertebrae.

Anatomy: The pharynx (throat) is a funnel-shaped muscular tube about 5-in long that begins at the internal nares and extends to the level of the cricoid cartilage, the inferior-most part of the larynx (Figure 1-1a).

Pharyngeal wall: The pharyngeal wall is formed from skeletal muscle, the superior, middle, and inferior constrictor muscles, and is lined with mucous membrane (non-keratinized stratified squamous) that is continuous with that of the mouth and nasal cavity.

Nasopharynx: The pharynx is divided into three portions: the uppermost portion, the nasopharynx lies posterior to the nasal cavity and extends to the plane of the soft palate. Opening into the nasopharynx are the two Eustachian (auditory) tubes from the middle ears.

Oropharynx: The middle portion of the pharynx, the oropharynx, lies posterior to the oral cavity. It extends from the soft palate to the level of the hyoid bone. The fauces is the opening from the mouth into the oropharynx.

Laryngopharynx: The lowermost portion of the pharynx, called thelaryngopharynx, becomes continuous with the opening of the esophagus posteriorly and the opening of the trachea anteriorly.

Function: The pharynx functions as a passageway for air and food and provides a resonating chamber for voice production.

Larynx

Location: The larynx (voice box) is a short passageway that connects the pharynx with the trachea. It lies in the midline of the neck anterior to vertebrae C4-C6.

Anatomy: The wall of the larynx is composed of nine cartilages placed in the shape of a box. The largest, the thyroid cartilage, forms the anterior wall of the larynx (Adam's apple). The cricoid cartilage, lying just posterior to the thyroid cartilage, forms a complete ring about the lower end of the larynx and is attached to the first ring of cartilage in the trachea.

Epiglottis: The epiglottis, one of the nine cartilages of the larynx, sits atop the box like a leaf, the stem of which is attached to the thyroid cartilage. The "leaf" portion of the cartilage is unattached and free to cover the anterior opening of the larynx, the glottis (Figure 1-2).

Swallowing: During the swallowing reflex, the larynx is elevated by skeletal muscle so that it is pulled up against the epiglottis. This prevents aspiration of food or drink. The epiglottis does not move down to cover the glottis.

Laryngospasm: When anything other than air touches the mucous membrane of the larynx, a cough reflex is initiated. The reflex causes us to cough so that the material is expelled. At the same time, reflex closure of the glottis occurs. This is called laryngospasm and explains why it is often hard to talk after choking.

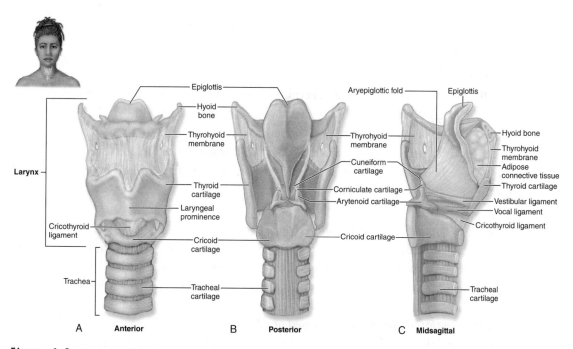

Figure 1-2 • Anatomy of the larynx.
Reproduced with permission from McKinley M, O'Loughlin VD. *Human Anatomy,* 2nd ed. 2008. New York: Copyright © McGraw-Hill Education. All rights reserved. Page 752.

Mucous membrane: The mucous membrane within the larynx is lined with ciliated pseudostratified epithelium and forms two pairs of folds. The upper pair of folds is called the ventricular folds (false vocal cords) and the lower pair of folds is the vocal folds (true vocal cords). The space between the vocal folds is the glottis. These are the anatomical features we are looking for when intubating (Figure 1-1b).

Voice production: Voice production occurs when the cartilages of the larynx are moved by skeletal muscles so that the true vocal cords are tightened or loosened. Air is then pushed past them in gusts. This causes the vocal cords to vibrate and make sounds. Sounds from the vibrating vocal folds are then modified by the pharynx, nasal cavity, paranasal sinuses, cheeks, teeth, and tongue to produce the sounds that we recognize.

Trachea

Location: The trachea (windpipe) is a tubular passageway for air about 5-in long and 1 in in diameter. It is located anterior to the esophagus and extends from the base of the larynx to the level of T5, where it divides into the primary bronchi.

Wall: The wall of the trachea is composed of four layers:

- Mucosa

- Submucosa

- Cartilage

- Adventitia

Mucosa/submucosa: The tracheal mucosa is ciliated pseudostratified epithelium with goblet cells (commonly called the respiratory epithelium). Beneath this is a submucosa of connective tissue and mucous glands.

Cartilage: The third layer of the tracheal wall is formed of 16-20 C-shaped rings of hyaline cartilage that are arranged horizontally and stacked atop one another (Figure 1-3).

Describe the open part of the C-shaped ring?
The open part of the "C" faces the esophagus. It is bridged by elastic connective tissue and smooth muscle fibers called the trachealis. This arrangement allows for the distention of the esophagus during swallowing (see Figure 1-3).

Describe the closed part of the C-shaped ring?
The solid portions of the cartilage rings are bridged by a dense connective tissue. This arrangement provides a rigid support so that the tracheal wall does not collapse inward and obstruct the air flow (think about a vacuum cleaner hose).

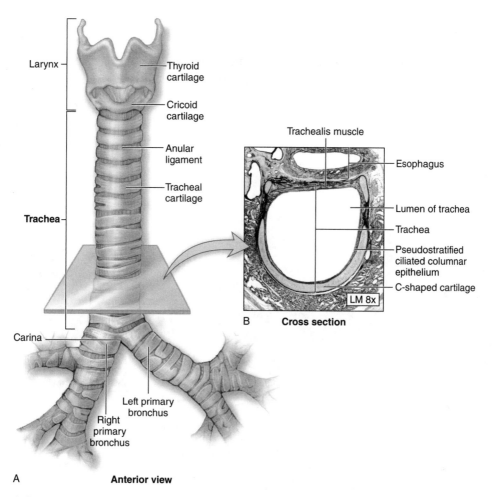

Figure 1-3 • Upper airway cross section.
Reproduced with permission from McKinley M, O'Loughlin VD. *Human Anatomy*, 2nd ed. 2008. New York: Copyright ©
McGraw-Hill Education. All rights reserved. Page 755.

Adventitia: The outermost coat of the trachea is an adventitia, a connective tissue layer that binds the trachea down within the neck.

Bronchi

Primary bronchi: At the level of T5, the trachea divides into the right and left primary bronchi, each of which then enters its respective lung. The right primary bronchus is more vertical, shorter, and wider than the left. As a result, most aspirated objects tend to enter the right bronchus (Figure 1-4).

Bronchial divisions: Immediately upon entering the lungs, the primary bronchi divide into smaller secondary (lobar) bronchi (three on the right and two

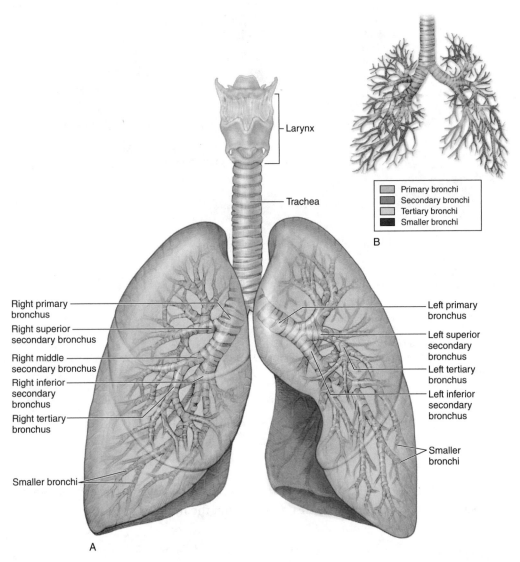

Primary bronchi
Secondary bronchi
Tertiary bronchi
Smaller bronchi

Larynx

Trachea

Right primary bronchus

Right superior secondary bronchus

Right middle secondary bronchus

Right inferior secondary bronchus

Right tertiary bronchus

Smaller bronchi

Left primary bronchus

Left superior secondary bronchus

Left tertiary bronchus

Left inferior secondary bronchus

Smaller bronchi

A

B

Figure 1-4 • Bronchial divisions.
Reproduced with permission from McKinley M, O'Loughlin VD. *Human Anatomy,* 2nd ed. 2008. New York: Copyright © McGraw-Hill Education. All rights reserved. Page 756.

on the left). The secondary bronchi divide further to form tertiary (segmental) bronchi (10 on the right and 8 on the left); see Figure 1-4.

Bronchioles: Tertiary bronchi continue to divide, forming bronchioles, which divide to form smaller and smaller ones, eventually forming the terminal bronchioles. Terminal bronchioles conduct air into respiratory bronchioles, which give rise to alveolar ducts, alveolar sacs, and finally the alveoli, the final gas exchange structures of the lungs (see Figure 1-4).

Histological changes: As the bronchial tree branches, three major anatomical changes occur in the: (1) cartilage, (2) epithelium, and (3) smooth muscle.

- The C-shaped rings of cartilage give way to irregular plates of cartilage around the secondary and tertiary bronchi, and then no cartilage at all around the bronchioles.

- The epithelium of the bronchial tree changes as follows: ciliated pseudostratified epithelium with goblet cells, ciliated cuboidal with goblet cells, ciliated cuboidal, cuboidal, at the alveolar sacs, simple squamous.

- As cartilage decreases, the circular smooth muscle in the bronchial wall increases. This muscle is controlled by the autonomic nervous system. Increased sympathetic outflow causes bronchodilation, while parasympathetic outflow causes bronchoconstriction. This is particularly effective at the bronchiolar level.

Lungs

Location: The lungs are paired, cone-shaped organs lying within the thoracic cavity. They are separated from each other by the heart and other structures in the mediastinum.

Pleura: Two layers of serous membrane, called the pleurae or pleural membrane, enclose and protect each lung. The outer layer, the parietal pleura, is attached to the inside of the thoracic wall. The inner layer, the visceral pleura, is intimately attached to the outer surface of each lung.

Pleural cavity: Between the two layers is a potential space called the pleural cavity which contains a small amount of serous fluid. The pleural cavity is considered a potential space because it is normally not present. In other words, the parietal and visceral pleurae are closely applied to one another with no real space between them.

Pleural fluid: Pleural fluid, created by the cells of the pleurae, serves as a lubricant to reduce friction between the two membranes as the lungs move. In addition, a negative pressure is created between the two layers, so that the

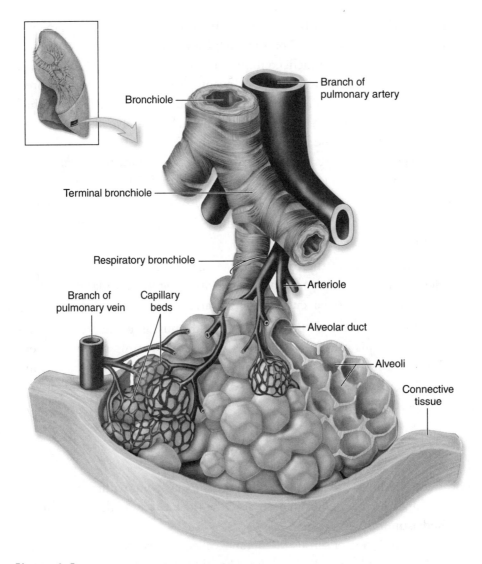

Figure 1-5 • Lower airway anatomy.
Reproduced with permission from McKinley M, O'Loughlin VD. *Human Anatomy*, 2nd ed. 2008.
New York: Copyright © McGraw-Hill Education. All rights reserved. Page 758.

parietal and visceral pleurae are held tightly against one another (like two panes of glass with water between them).

Function of the pleura: The parietal pleura is attached to the inside of the thoracic wall. Since there is negative pressure in the pleural cavity, the visceral pleura is "pulled" out against the parietal pleura (leaving only a potential space between them). Visceral pleura are attached to the outer surface of the lungs and the lungs are elastic, so the lungs are also stretched out, filling the thoracic cavity.

Gross Anatomy of the Lungs

Lobes and fissures   Location: The lungs extend from the diaphragm inferiorly (base of the lungs) to just above the clavicles (apex) and lie against the ribs anteriorly, posteriorly, and laterally.

Hilus: On the medial surface of lung there is an indentation called the hilus. It is through the hilus that the primary bronchus, pulmonary artery, bronchial artery, pulmonary veins, autonomic nerves, and lymphatics enter and exit the lungs.

Right lung: The right lung is divided into three lobes (superior, middle, and inferior) by the horizontal fissure and the oblique fissure. Each lobe receives a secondary bronchus.

Left lung: The left lung is divided into two lobes (superiorand inferior) by the oblique fissure. Each lobe receives a secondary bronchus.

Lobules and the Alveolar-Capillary (Respiratory) Membrane

Lobules: Each lung is further subdivided by tertiary bronchi into broncho-pulmonary segments, each of which is divided into lobules by terminal bronchioles. Each lobule is wrapped in elastic tissue and contains a lymphatic vessel, pulmonary arteriole, bronchial arteriole, pulmonary venule, and a terminal bronchiole.

Alveolus: Terminal bronchioles give rise to respiratory bronchioles, alveolar ducts, alveolar sacs, and finally individual alveoli. An alveolus is a cup-shaped out-pouching of the alveolar duct epithelium, formed of two types of simple squamous cells resting on a very thin basement membrane.

Type I alveolar cell: Type I alveolar cells (squamous pulmonary epithelial cells) form the continuous lining of the alveolus and are the cells across which gases diffuse between the lungs and the blood (external respiration) (Figure 1-6).

Type II alveolar cell: Type II alveolar (septal) cells are found scattered among the others and function to secrete an alveolar fluid that keeps the alveolar cells moist. One component of this fluid is surfactant, a phospholipid (Figure 1-6).

Surfactant acts to lower the surface tension of alveolar fluid, since the attractive forces between water molecules would cause the alveoli to collapse. It is not created until late in the pregnancy. This is why premature infants have great difficulty breathing.

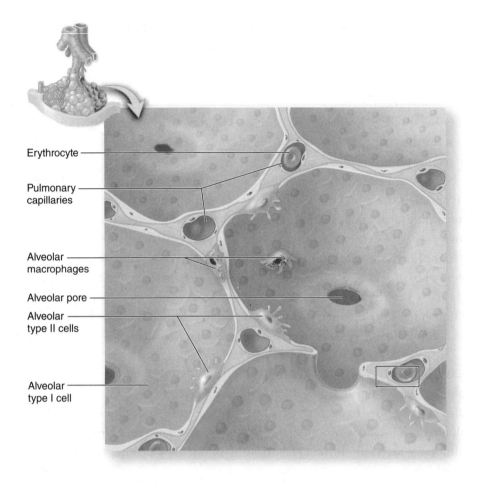

Figure 1-6 • Alveolar anatomy.
Reproduced with permission from McKinley M, O'Loughlin VD. *Human Anatomy*, 2nd ed. 2008.
New York: Copyright © McGraw-Hill Education. All rights reserved. Page 759.

What Went Wrong?

Premature babies are at risk for respiratory distress at birth. Immature lung tissue can make breathing difficult for premature babies. Respiratory distress most often affects premature babies born before 34 weeks. Approximately 10% of premature babies experience some degree of distress.

Surfactant deficiency in premature infants is a serious, possibly life-threatening condition that results in respiratory distress and pulmonary failure if left untreated. Pulmonary surfactant is a naturally occurring slippery substance made of phospholipids and proteins; it lines the alveoli, or air sacs, in the lungs and reduces surface tension. This serves to help the lungs function properly and prevents alveoli collapse. Infants suffering from surfactant deficiency do not have enough open alveoli to draw in sufficient air.

Newborns without enough pulmonary surfactants are diagnosed with respiratory distress syndrome (RDS). The symptoms may include: rapid, shallow breathing; flared nostrils showing physical strain in breathing; sharp pulling in of the chest below and between the ribs; wheezing and grunting as the body tries to retain air; and bluish or pale grey coloring of the skin due to lack of oxygen. Infants with surfactant deficiency may also experience apnea.

Premature infants are most prone to RDS; more than half of those born before 28 weeks of pregnancy are diagnosed with the condition. This is because pulmonary surfactants began to be produced around 24 to 36 weeks of gestation. Infants born prematurely have not developed adequate levels of surfactant and therefore need assistance in breathing for the first few days.

Treatment options for surfactant deficiency may include all or several of the following:

- Artificial surfactant therapy: directly administering surfactant to the infant's lungs. Usually one dose is enough, but some infants require repeated treatment over the course of 2 to 3 days.

- Mechanical ventilator: assists the infant in breathing by pushing air into the lungs through a breathing tube.

- Nasal continuous positive airway pressure (NCPAP): assists in breathing by continuously pushing air into the lungs through small tubes inserted into the nose.

- Extra oxygen: infants with respiratory distress require a higher level of oxygen.

Alveolar macrophage: This is a third type of cell (dust cell) that wanders through the interstitial spaces of the lungs, removing foreign particles and other debris.

So what is the respiratory membrane (alveolar-capillary membrane)?

The exchange of respiratory gases between the lungs and blood takes place by diffusion across the alveolar and capillary walls. Collectively, these layers are called the alveolar-capillary (respiratory) membrane.

The respiratory membrane consists of three layers:

1. Alveolar epithelial cell
2. Fused basement membranes of alveolar epithelial cell and capillary endothelial cell
3. Capillary endothelial cell

How does its structure enhance gas diffusion?

The membrane is very thin, averaging about 0.5 microns in thickness. This allows rapid diffusion of the respiratory gases. Along with this, the lungs contain some 300 million alveoli, providing an immense surface area for gas diffusion (750 sq. ft.-about the size of a racquetball court).

Blood Supply to the Lungs

Pulmonary artery: The pulmonary artery carries deoxygenated blood from the right ventricle to the lung. Each time the bronchial tree branches, so does this artery. The result is that each lobule has its own branch of the pulmonary artery carrying deoxygenated blood for gas exchange.

Bronchial artery: The bronchial artery branches from the descending aorta as it passes the hilus of each lung. It supplies oxygenated blood to the walls of the bronchial tree.

Pulmonary vein: The pulmonary veins are formed as the capillaries of the pulmonary artery and bronchial artery merge. The branches of the veins follow the bronchial tree back to the hilus where normally two pulmonary veins from each lung emerge to carry all venous blood back to the left atrium (oxygenated blood). There are no bronchial veins.

Physiology of Respiration

What is the principal purpose of respiration?

The principal purpose of respiration is to supply the cells of the body with oxygen while removing carbon dioxide formed by cellular metabolism.

There are three processes needed to accomplish this task.

1. Pulmonary ventilation
   - Inspiration
   - Expiration
2. External respiration
3. Internal respiration

Pulmonary Ventilation

Pulmonary ventilation (breathing) is the process by which gases are moved between the atmosphere and the alveoli of the lungs (inspiration and expiration). The flow of air between the two occurs because a pressure gradient is created. When atmospheric pressure is greater than intrapulmonic pressure, air flows from the atmosphere into the lungs to fill the alveoli. When intrapulmonic pressure is greater than atmospheric pressure, air flows from the alveoli, through the bronchial tree, and into the atmosphere.

Inspiration

Breathing in is called inspiration (inhalation). Just before it occurs, air pressure within the lungs (intrapulmonic pressure) equals atmospheric pressure. For air to flow into the lungs from the atmosphere, intrapulmonic air pressure must become less than atmospheric air pressure. To accomplish this, the volume (size) of the lungs is increased. To understand how this reduces intrapulmonic pressure, one must understand the Boyle's law—the pressure of a gas in a closed container is inversely proportional to the volume of the container. In other words, if the size of a closed container is increased, the air pressure within decreases; if the size of the container is decreased, the air pressure within increases. If you assume that the respiratory system is a closed container, then increasing the size of the lungs causes intrapulmonic pressure to decrease. When intrapulmonic pressure becomes less than atmospheric pressure, then air flows down its pressure gradient into the lungs. In order for inspiration to occur, the lungs must first expand. The first step in this process involves contraction of the respiratory skeletal muscles, the diaphragm, and 11 pairs of external intercostal muscles (Figure 1-7).

The dome-shaped diaphragm, the most important muscle of respiration, is innervated by the phrenic nerves (C3-C5). In response to stimulation, the diaphragm contracts pulling down and toward the abdominal cavity. At the same time the 11 pairs of external intercostal muscles, innervated by T1-T11, contract, pulling the rib cage up and out. As a result of these muscular movements, the length of the thoracic cavity, as well as its anteroposterior diameter, is increased, so that thoracic volume increases. Movement of the thoracic walls carries the

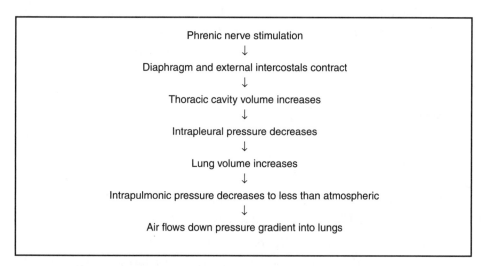

Phrenic nerve stimulation
↓
Diaphragm and external intercostals contract
↓
Thoracic cavity volume increases
↓
Intrapleural pressure decreases
↓
Lung volume increases
↓
Intrapulmonic pressure decreases to less than atmospheric
↓
Air flows down pressure gradient into lungs

Figure 1-7 • Summary of inspiration.
Reproduced with permission from Human Anatomy, McKinley, Michael and Valerie Dean O'Loughlin, 2nd ed.

parietal pleura away from the visceral pleura, resulting in increased intrapleural volume, and therefore decreased intrapleural pressure. As a result, the visceral pleura follow the parietal pleura, stretching the lungs to fill the increased volume of the thorax. This, in turn, increases intrapulmonic volume and the intrapulmonic pressure decreases. When intrapulmonic pressure becomes less than the atmospheric pressure, air flows into the lungs and continues until the two pressures are equal. Inspiration is said to be an active process since skeletal muscle contraction is required. Normally, only the diaphragm and external intercostals are used, but there are accessoryinspiratorymuscles for specialized inspirations (deep breathing, yawning, etc).

Expiration

Expiration (exhalation), or breathing out, is considered a passive process, because no skeletal muscle contraction is necessary during normal breathing at rest. Expiration is also achieved by a pressure gradient, but in this case it is reversed, and is dependent upon two factors:

1. Elastic recoil of the lungs after they were stretched during inspiration.
2. The inward pull of surface tension due to the film of alveolar fluid.

Expiration begins when inspiratory muscles relax, allowing the thoracic cavity to return to its resting volume. In addition, elastic recoil and surface tension tend to exert inward forces on the lungs, making lung volume decrease. Boyle's law states that decreasing volume causes an increase in air pressure, so intrapulmonic pressure rises. When intrapulmonic pressure exceeds atmospheric pressure, air flows down its pressure gradient, back into the atmosphere from the lungs. There are accessory muscles of expiration (internal intercostals, anterior abdominal wall muscles) which can cause forceful expirations (coughing, sneezing, laughing, etc) (Figure 1-8).

Compliance

Compliance refers to the ease with which the lungs and thoracic wall can be expanded.

- Elasticity of the lungs and surface tension in the alveoli
- Compliance is decreased with any condition that:
  1. destroys the lung tissue (emphysema).
  2. fills the lungs with fluid (pneumonia).
  3. produces a deficiency of surfactant (premature birth, near-drowning).
  4. Interferes with lung expansion (pneumothorax).

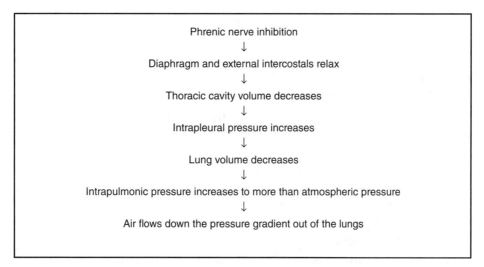

Phrenic nerve inhibition
↓
Diaphragm and external intercostals relax
↓
Thoracic cavity volume decreases
↓
Intrapleural pressure increases
↓
Lung volume decreases
↓
Intrapulmonic pressure increases to more than atmospheric pressure
↓
Air flows down the pressure gradient out of the lungs

Figure 1-8 • Expiration.

Pulmonary Air Volumes and Capacities

Clinical respiration: In clinical respiration, the word respiration (ventilation) refers to one inspiration and one expiration. A normal resting adult, averages 12 respirations per minute, and moves about 6 liters of air into and out of the lungs. These 6 liters of air (average) can be divided into several different pulmonary volumes and capacities, which can be seen with a spirogram.

Tidal volume (TV): Tidal volume = approximately 500 mL. This is the air which moves into the respiratory passages with each resting inspiration, then out with each resting expiration.

Anatomical dead space: Of the 500 mL TV, only about 350 mL reaches the alveoli for gas exchange. The other 150 mL fills the conducting portion of the system where gas exchange cannot occur. This area is called the anatomical dead space.

Minute volume: The total air taken in during 1 minute is the minute volume of respiration (MVR). It is determined by multiplying TV by breaths per minute.

Inspiratory reserve volume (IRV): Inspiratory reserve volume = 3,100 mL. This is the volume of air that can forcefully be inspired after a normal tidal volume inspiration.

Expiratory reserve volume (ERV): Expiratory reserve volume= 1,200 mL. This is the volume of air that can be forcefully expired after a normal tidal volume expiration.

Residual volume (RV): Residual volume = 1,200 mL. This is the volume of air that remains in the lungs even after a forceful expiration. It is established with the first breath at birth and is replenished with each breath. Its purpose is to ensure that gas exchange with the blood occurs 100% of the time.

Vital capacity: Vital capacity = 4,800 mL. This is the sum of TV + IRV + ERV. It represents the total volume of air that can be moved forcibly into and out of the lungs.

Exchanges of Oxygen and Carbon Dioxide

At birth, as soon as the lungs fill with air, oxygen starts to flow down its concentration gradient from the alveoli, into the blood, into the interstitial fluid, and finally into body cells. At the same time, carbon dioxide diffuses in the other direction, from the body cells to the interstitial fluid, into the blood, and finally into the alveoli, again following its concentration gradient.

Movement of these gases between fluid compartments is according to which of the gas laws?

Movement of these gases between fluid compartments is according to Dalton's law.

Dalton's Law

According to Dalton's law, each gas in a mixture of gases exerts its own pressure as if all the other gases were not present.

Partial pressure: The pressure of a specific gas in a mixture of gases is known as its partial pressure (p). The total pressure of a mixture of gases is the sum of the partial pressures.

What are the pressures associated with atmospheric air at sea level?

The pressures are as follows:

Atmospheric air pressure = 760 mm Hg
Nitrogen = 597 mm Hg +
Oxygen = 160 mm Hg +
Carbon dioxide = 0.3 mm Hg +
Water vapor = 2.7 mm Hg +

In which direction will oxygen diffuse in the case below? Why?

The partial pressures determine the direction in which oxygen will diffuse. Since body cells constantly use oxygen during energy production, diffusion never reaches equilibrium, and oxygen constantly moves to the cells (see Figure 1-9).

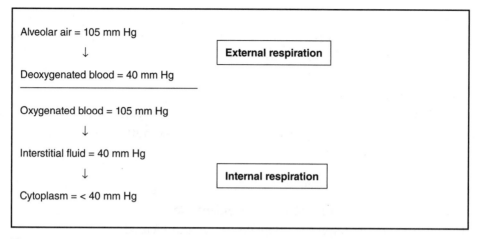

Figure 1-9 • Diffusion of oxygen during respiration.

In which direction will carbon dioxide diffuse? Why

The partial pressure determines the direction in which carbon dioxide will diffuse. Since body cells constantly make carbon dioxide during energy production, diffusion never reaches equilibrium, and carbon dioxide constantly moves from the cells (see Figure 1-10).

Physiology of External (Pulmonary) Respiration

External (pulmonary) respiration is the movement of oxygen and carbon dioxide between alveoli of the lungs and the blood of pulmonary capillaries. It

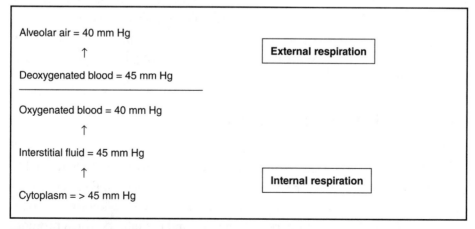

Figure 1-10 • Diffusion of carbon dioxide during respiration.

results in the conversion of deoxygenated blood to oxygenated blood for return to the left side of the heart. At the same time, it results in the loss of carbon dioxide from the blood into the alveoli, so it can be breathed away.

How much diffusion occurs?

Diffusion of each gas occurs 100% of the time and not just until equilibrium. Pulmonary blood flow is continuous rather than intermittent because of pulmonary capillaries, and therefore pulmonary blood passes several alveoli before passing out of the lung.

What factors are external respiration dependent upon?

The rate of external respiration depends upon four factors:

1. Partial pressure differences between the gases

2. Surface area for diffusion

3. Diffusion distance

4. Breathing rate and depth

Physiology of Internal (Tissue) Respiration

Internal (tissue) respiration is the exchange of oxygen and carbon dioxide between the blood of systemic capillaries and interstitial fluid and therefore body cells. Because cells constantly use oxygen and produce carbon dioxide, there is a constant diffusion gradient delivering fresh oxygen to and removing the carbon dioxide from the tissues.

How much diffusion occurs?

At rest, only about 25% of total oxygen in the blood is delivered to the tissues. This amount is sufficient to support the cells and give a large reserve in case of cardiovascular or respiratory failure. As with external respiration, equilibrium of the gases is never reached because the blood flow through the systemic capillaries is continuous.

Transport of Oxygen and Carbon Dioxide

Oxygen

Oxygen (O_2) (98.5%) is transported in chemical combination with hemoglobin (Hb) within RBCs. The other 1.5% is dissolved in the plasma. Each Hb molecule binds to four molecules of O_2 in a freely reversible reaction to form oxyhemoglobin. It is therefore important to understand the factors which promote

O_2 binding and dissociation from Hb. The most important factor that determines how much O_2 binds to Hb is the partial pressure of oxygen. When reduced Hb is completely converted to oxyhemoglobin, it is said to be fully saturated. When Hb is in a mixture of reduced Hb and oxyhemoglobin, it is said to be partially saturated. The percent saturation of hemoglobin is the percent of oxyhemoglobin to total Hb. The relationship that exists between percent saturation of Hb and the partial pressure of oxygen is shown by the oxygen-hemoglobin dissociation curve. When oxygen partial pressure is 80-100 mm Hg, Hb is >90% saturated. Thus, in the lungs, where oxygen partial pressure is high, blood picks up nearly a full load of oxygen. In the tissues, where oxygen partial pressure is lower, Hb does not hold oxygen as well, so O_2 is released for diffusion to the cells. At a partial pressure of 40, Hb is only about 75% saturated. Thus about 25% of blood oxygen is liberated to the tissues. In active tissues, where the oxygen partial pressure may be less than 40 mm Hg (i.e. contracting skeletal muscle) a large percentage of O_2 is released to the cells.

Carbon Dioxide

Other factors that affect the saturation of Hb with oxygen include pH (acidity), partial pressure of carbon dioxide (CO_2) (which is related to pH), and temperature. In an acidic environment (pH <7.4), Hb's affinity for oxygen is reduced and O_2 splits more readily from Hb (dissociation curve shifts to the right). This means that more O_2 is supplied to the tissues. This is known as the Bohr effect. It occurs because hydrogen ions bind to Hb and change its molecular structure, thereby decreasing Hb's oxygen-carrying ability. Since active tissues generate acid (hydrogen ions), this is another mean to ensure that adequate O_2 is delivered to the tissues to support their activity. Active tissues also create more CO_2 than resting tissues. Increased CO_2 promotes increased formation of hydrogen ions, so there is a decreased pH. The net effect is a shift in the dissociation curve to the right (the Bohr effect, in essence), so that more O_2 is supplied to the active tissues. Temperature also affects Hb saturation: as temperature increases, the dissociation curve is shifted to the right. Active tissues create heat; this is yet another way to ensure adequate oxygen delivery to an active tissue.

Name the three methods by which CO_2 is transported in the blood. Give the percentage for each.

The three methods by which CO_2 is transported in the blood are as follows:

1. Dissolved in plasma (7%)
2. Bound in Hb (carbaminohemoglobin) (23%)
3. As bicarbonate ion (70%)

Describe the relationship between CO_2, H^+ and HCO_3^-.

The reaction that creates bicarbonate ion from carbon dioxide is as follows:

$$CO_2 + H_2O \longleftrightarrow H_2CO_3 \longleftrightarrow H^+ + HCO_3^-$$

This is a freely reversible reaction that is catalyzed by the enzyme carbonic anhydrase in the RBC cytoplasm. In venous blood, where pCO_2 is high, the reaction is shifted to the right, so that H^+ ions and HCO_3^- are formed. The H^+ ions bind to Hb (Bohr Effect) so that oxygen is released. The HCO_3^- diffuses into the plasma (in exchange for chloride ions—the chloride shift) and is carried to the lungs in the deoxygenated blood. In pulmonary blood, dissolved CO_2 and that bound to Hb leave the blood and diffuse into the alveoli. Since the oxygen partial pressure is high in the lungs, Hb releases its bound H and binds to oxygen. The increased H^+ concentration causes the reaction to shift to the left so that CO_2 and H_2O are reformed. The CO_2 diffuses from the RBC into the plasma and thence into the alveoli. This relationship between CO_2 and H^+ ions (and therefore pH) is very important in the use of the respiratory mechanisms when compensating for pH imbalances and helps explain how respiratory disease leads to pH imbalance.

Where does this reaction take place?

$$CO_2 + H_2O \leftarrow H_2CO_3 \leftarrow H^+ + HCO_3^-$$

The reaction in this direction occurs in the lungs because in the lungs, increased oxygen partial pressure causes Hb to release hydrogen ions and bind to O_2. Increased hydrogen ions cause the reaction to shift to the left so that CO_2 is reformed. It then diffuses into the alveoli so it can be breathed away.

What is the fate of carbon dioxide, hydrogen ions, and bicarbonate ions?

Carbon dioxide diffuses into the alveoli and breathed away. Hydrogen ions are released from Hb into RBC cytoplasm, and then used in the generation of CO_2 and water. Bicarbonate ions diffuse into RBC from plasma, then used in the generation of CO_2 and water.

Where does this reaction take place?

$$CO_2 + H_2O \rightarrow H_2CO_3 \rightarrow H^+ + HCO_3^-$$

Seventy percent of CO_2 is funneled into the reaction, causing it to shift to the right. This leads to the formation of H^+ ions and HCO_3^- ions. Hydrogen ions bind to Hb, causing oxygen to be released, and the HCO_3^- diffuses into the plasma in exchange for chloride ions.

Carbon dioxide diffuses from tissues into the blood for transport to the lungs. Hydrogen ions bind to Hb, causing the release of O_2 (Bohr effect) Bicarbonate ions diffuse into plasma in exchange for chloride ions (chloride shift).

Control of Respiration

Nervous Control: Medullary Rhythmicity Area

Mechanisms must exist that match respiratory effort with metabolic demands as we move from states of relative inactivity to states of great activity. The respiratory center, jointly located in the medulla and pons of the brain stem, transmits nervous impulses to the respiratory muscles. It is divided into three

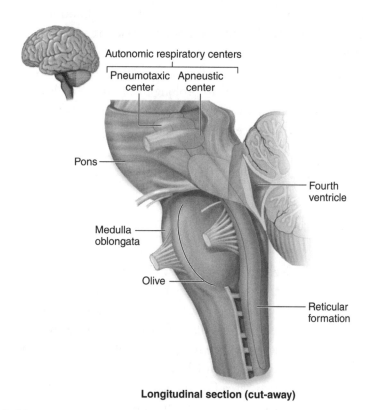

Longitudinal section (cut-away)

Figure 1-11 • Autonomic respiratory center.
Source: McKinley, Michael and Valerie Dean O'Loughlin. *Human Anatomy,* 2nd ed. Figure 15.20A, page 465.

portions; the medullary rhythmicity area functions in the control of the basic rhythm of breathing. It is further subdivided into two separate but interconnected groups of neurons: an inspiratory area and an expiratory area. At rest, inspiration is an active process that requires about 2 seconds, while expiration is passive and requires about 3 seconds (12 breaths per minute). Inspiratory neurons generate action potential automatically that are transmitted to the respiratory muscles. After 2 seconds, this ends, the respiratory muscles relax, and expiration begins. During times of high ventilation rate, the inspiratory neurons fire more often and stimulate the accessory muscles of inspiration. They also stimulate the expiratory neurons so that the muscles of forced expiration can be stimulated.

Pneumotaxic and Apneustic Area

Pneumotaxic area: The pneumotaxic area, a group of neurons in the pons, transmits inhibitory messages to the inspiratory area. The effect is to limit inspiration before the lungs become too full of air. This limits the duration of inspiration and facilitates expiration. When the pneumotaxic area is more active, the breathing rate is faster.

Apneustic area: The apneustic area, a second group of neurons in the pons, stimulates the inspiratory neurons to prolong inspiration and limit expiration. This action occurs when the pneumotaxic area is inactive; when the pneumotaxic area is active, its influence overrides the activity of the apneustic area.

Regulation of Respiratory Center Activity

- Cortical influence
- Inflation reflex
- Chemical regulation

Cortical influences: The cerebral cortex, as well as the hypothalamus and limbic system, have input into the respiratory center, so that we have some conscious control over breathing (holding our breath, for example).

Inflation reflex: Located in the walls of the bronchial tree are stretch receptors which are stimulated when the lungs are inflated, initiating the inflation (Hering-Breuer) reflex. Action potentials from these receptors inhibit the inspiratory area and the apneustic area (via the vagus nerve). This allows expiration to begin. Once the lungs are deflated, inspiration is free to occur again.

Chemical influences: The influence of higher brain neurons is limited however, by the buildup of CO_2 and hydrogen ions in the blood, since they directly

A stimulus or stress disrupts homeostasis by causing an increase in arterial CO_2 or a decrease in pH or O_2.

↓

RECEPTORS: Chemoreceptive neurons of the medulla and chemoreceptors in the aortic and carotid bodies respond to changes and direct nerve impulses to the control center.

↓

CONTROL CENTER: The inspiratory neurons of the medulla receives the sensory input, interpret its meaning and generate impulses which pass to the effectors.

↓

EFFECTORS: The diaphragm, external intercostals, and other muscles of inspiration are stimulated to contract more frequently and more forcefully, resulting in hyperventilation.

↓

RESPONSES: RETURN TO HOMEOSTASIS: Hyperventilation results in a decrease in arterial blood carbon dioxide, an increase in pH, and an increase in blood oxygen content. This returns the blood to homeostasis.

Figure 1-12 • Regulation of respiration.

stimulate the inspiratory neurons. In other words, you can only hold your breath so long, because inspiratory neurons will force inspiration when there is a high concentration of CO_2 or H^+.

The ultimate goal of the respiratory system is to maintain proper levels of O_2 and CO_2 in the blood. The respiratory system is sensitive to changes in either. In the medulla are neurons particularly sensitive to hydrogen ions. Located in the carotid arteries and aorta are chemoreceptors which constantly monitor arterial blood concentration of hydrogen, CO_2, and O_2. Too much hydrogen or CO_2, or too little O_2, results in reflex stimulation of the inspiratory area and therefore an increased respiratory rate (hyperventilation).

Too few hydrogen ions or too little CO_2 causes the inspiratory system to operate more slowly (hypoventilation), and allows the levels to rise, thus returning to normal.

When an arterial $pO_2 = 50$ mm Hg or less, inspiratory neurons become hypoxic (too little O_2) and cannot function normally. As a result, there is decreased stimulation to inspire, resulting in less arterial oxygen. The continued decrease in arterial oxygen causes the neurons to be even less active. This becomes a positive feedback cycle and results in death without clinical intervention (see Figures 1-12 and 1-13).

A stimulus or stress disrupts homeostasis by causing a decrease in arterial-oxygen below 50 mm Hg.

↓

RECEPTORS: Chemoreceptive neurons of the medulla suffer hypoxia, resulting in the output of fewer nerve impulses.

↓

CONTROL CENTER: The inspiratory neurons of the medulla suffer hypoxia, resulting the output of fewer nerve impulses to the inspiratory muscles.

↓

EFFECTORS: The diaphragm, external intercostals, and other muscles of inspiration are stimulated to contract less frequently and less forcefully, resulting in hypoventilation.

↓

RESPONSES: NO RETURN TO HOMEOSTASIS: Hypoventilation results in a decrease in arterial blood oxygen content, causing greater hypoxia. This results in positive feedback and more disruption of homeostasis.

Figure 1-13 • Dysfunction of respiration.

REVIEW QUESTIONS

1. **The exchange of gases between blood and cells is called**

   A. pulmonary ventilation.
   B. internal respiration.
   C. external respiration.
   D. cellular respiration.

Correct answer is b.

2. **Which of the following does not belong to the conducting portion of the respiratory system?**

   A. Alveoli
   B. Bronchioles
   C. Nose
   D. Pharynx

Correct answer is a.

3. **The structure which closes off the larynx is the**

   A. glottis.
   B. Adam's apple.
   C. epiglottis.
   D. vocal cords.

Correct answer is c.

4. **Which of the following describes the correct order of structures in the respiratory passageways?**

   A. Pharynx, trachea, larynx, bronchi, bronchioles
   B. Larynx, pharynx, trachea, bronchioles, bronchi
   C. Trachea, pharynx, larynx, bronchi, bronchioles
   D. Pharynx, larynx, trachea, bronchi, bronchioles

Correct answer is d.

5. **The exchange of gases occurs in the**

   A. trachea.
   B. bronchioles.
   C. alveoli.
   D. bronchus.

Correct answer is c.

6. **The volume of air that can be exhaled after normal exhalation is the**

   A. tidal volume.
   B. residual volume.
   C. inspiratory reserve volume.
   D. expiratory reserve volume.

Correct answer is d.

7. **The volume of air in a normal breath is called**

   A. total lung capacity.
   B. vital capacity.
   C. tidal volume.
   D. residual volume.

Correct answer is c.

8. Gas exchange in the lungs happens by the process of
    A. osmosis.
    B. diffusion.
    C. exocytosis.
    D. active transport.

Correct answer is b.

9. Most oxygen in the blood is transported
    A. as gas dissolved in plasma.
    B. as oxyhemoglobin.
    C. as carboxyhemoglobin.
    D. as bicarbonate.

Correct answer is b.

10. The primary chemical stimulus for breathing is the concentration of
    A. carbon monoxide in the blood.
    B. carbon dioxide in the blood.
    C. oxygen in the blood.
    D. carbonic acid in the blood.

Correct answer is b.

11. During inspiration, air is forced into the lungs by atmospheric pressure. Atmospheric air pressure is the pressure exerted by the air on all surfaces of the earth including our bodies. At sea level, it is equivalent to the pressure required to raise a column of mercury _____ mm Hg.
    A. 762
    B. 760
    C. 758
    D. 756

Correct answer is b.

12. During contraction of the diaphragm, as the diaphragm moves downward it results in a longer thoracic cavity. As a result, the intra-alveolar pressure is reduced to about _____ mm Hg.
    A. 762
    B. 760
    C. 758
    D. 756

Correct answer is c.

13. _____ states that gas volume is inversely proportional to pressure.

   A. Starling law
   B. Murphy's law
   C. Peter's law
   D. Boyle's law

Correct answer is d.

14. Tidal volume in an adult measures approximately _____ mL.

   A. 450
   B. 500
   C. 600
   D. 800

Correct answer is b.

15. The volume of air remaining in the lungs at all times is called _____.

   A. functional reserve volume
   B. vital capacity
   C. residual volume
   D. inspiratory capacity

Correct answer is c.

16. _____ _____ bronchus is wider, shorter, and runs more vertically than the _____ _____ bronchus as it passes directly to the hilum of the lung.

   A. Left main; right main
   B. Right main, left main
   C. Middle main, right main
   D. None of the above

   Correct answer is b.

17. The _____ main bronchus passes inferolaterally, inferior to the arch of the aorta and anterior to the esophagus.

   A. left
   B. right
   C. middle
   D. superior

Correct answer is a.

18. Each lung has _____ large pulmonary artery and _____ pulmonary veins draining blood from it.

   A. two; one
   B. three; one
   C. one; two
   D. one; one

Correct answer is c.

19. The _____ pleura covers the lungs and is adherent to all its surfaces, including the surfaces, including the surfaces within the horizontal and oblique fissures; it cannot be dissected from the lungs.

   A. visceral
   B. parietal
   C. cervical
   D. None of the above

Correct answer is a.

20. The _____ pleura line the pulmonary cavities, adhering to the thoracic wall, the mediastinum, and the diaphragm.

   A. visceral
   B. parietal
   C. cervical
   D. None of the above

Correct answer is b.

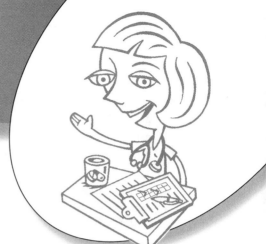

chapter 2

Acid-Base Balance, Blood Gas Analysis

LEARNING OBJECTIVES

At the end of this chapter, you will be able to:

1. Describe the physiology involved in the acid-base balance of the body.

2. Compare the roles of PaO_2, pH, $PaCO_2$, and bicarbonate in maintaining acid-base balance.

3. Discuss causes and treatments of respiratory acidosis, respiratory alkalosis, metabolic acidosis, and metabolic alkalosis.

4. Identify normal arterial blood gas (ABG) values and interpret the meaning of abnormal values.

5. Interpret the results of various ABG samples.

6. Identify the relationship between oxygen saturation and PaO_2 as it relates to the oxyhemoglobin dissociation curve.

7. Interpret the oxygenation state of a patient using the reported arterial blood gas PaO_2 value.

KEY TERMS

Acid-base balance
Arterial blood gas
Bicarbonate/carbonic acid-buffer system
Hemoglobin-buffer system
Metabolic acidosis

Metabolic alkalosis
Phosphate-buffer system
Physiological buffer systems
Protein-buffer system
Respiratory acidosis
Respiratory alkalosis

Scenario

A 44-year-old moderately dehydrated man was admitted with a 2-day history of acute severe diarrhea. He is now being transferred from a community hospital to a tertiary care medical center. Table 2-1 presents electrolyte results.

TABLE 2–1 Electrolyte Results			
134 Sodium	108 Chloride	31 BUN	124 Glucose
2.9 Potassium	16 Bicarbonate	1.5 Creatinine	

ABG: pH: 7.31 and pCO_2: 33 mm Hg
HCO_3 16 and pO_2 93 mm Hg

What is the acid-base disorder for this patient?

- Normal anion gap acidosis from diarrhea, or
- Elevated anion gap acidosis secondary to lactic acidosis as a result of hypovolemia and poor perfusion.

Introduction

Normal metabolic function can occur only if the composition of the body cells and their surrounding environment are kept relatively constant. Therefore, one of the most important functions of the body is the careful regulation of both fluid and electrolyte balance, and acid-base balance.

Disturbances in the acid-base balance of the body leads to cellular dysfunction and can seriously jeopardize a patient's life. Necessary metabolic activities can proceed only if the balance between acidic and basic substances in body fluids is kept within proper limits. The activities of virtually all the enzymes within the cells are to some extent pH-dependent.

Even more important is the pH dependence of the overall functioning of the body (ie, membrane transport processes and ionic states of all substances). In an acidic or basic environment, some chemical reactions are accelerated while others are slowed down and can even be stopped completely. It is, therefore, important to understand the mechanisms involved in maintaining the body's normal acid-base balance, and the consequences of acid-base disturbances.

Acid-base balance, is it really a balancing act?

The pH is a measurement of acidity or alkalinity of the blood. It is inversely proportional to the number of hydrogen ions (H^+) in the blood. The more H^+ present, the lower the pH will be. Likewise, the fewer H^+ present, the higher the pH will be. The pH of a solution is measured on a scale from 1 (very acidic) to 14 (very alkalotic). A liquid with a pH of 7, such as "pure" water, is neutral (neither acidic nor alkalotic).

The normal blood pH range is 7.35 to 7.45. For normal metabolism to take place, the body must maintain this narrow range at all times. When the pH is below 7.35, the blood is said to be *acidic.* Changes in body system functions that occur in an acidic state include a decrease in the force of cardiac contractions, a decrease in the vascular response to catecholamines, and a diminished response to the effects and actions of certain medications. When the pH is above 7.45, the blood is said to be *alkalotic.* An alkalotic state interferes with tissue oxygenation and normal neurological and muscular functioning. Significant changes in the blood pH above 7.8 or below 6.8 will interfere with cellular functioning, and if not treated, will lead to death (Figure 2-1).

How is the body able to self-regulate acid-base balance to maintain pH within the normal range?

It is accomplished using delicate buffer mechanisms between the respiratory and renal systems.

What Went Wrong?

For cardiopulmonary resuscitation (CPR), emphasis is on the importance of high-quality chest compressions (rate, depth, recoil), with minimum interruptions

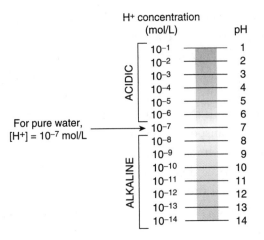

Figure 2-1 • pH scale.
Reproduced with permission from Barrett KE, Barman SM, Boitano S, Brooks HL, eds. *Ganong's Review of Medical Physiology.* 24th ed. 2012. New York: Copyright © McGraw-Hill Education. All rights reserved.

and early defibrillation when appropriate. In any case, drug delivery should not cause significant interruptions in these interventions. No drug has been definitively shown to improve survival to hospital discharge after cardiac arrest. However, evaluation of drugs is difficult after prolonged ischemia time, which minimizes the probability of survival.

The Physiological-Buffer Systems

An acid-base buffer is a chemical solution which prevents excessive change in pH (and H^+ concentration) when either acid or base is added to the solution. Specifically, a buffer is a mixture of either a weak acid and its alkali salt, or a weak base and its acid salt. In the body, the buffers of physiological importance are mixtures of weak acids and their alkali salts. If excess base is added to the solution, the weak acid part of the buffer reacts to neutralize it. Likewise if excess acid is added to the solution, the alkali salt part of the buffer reacts to neutralize it. In this way, the body's buffers can be regarded as chemical sponges, soaking up surplus H^+ or releasing them as required. The entire base that is available for immediate neutralization of acids produced by cell metabolism is in the form of buffer salts. Thus, it is only by the chemical action of these buffers that H^+ can be transported in the blood to the lungs and kidneys for excretion without the blood pH dropping drastically. The chemical action of the buffers occurs within a fraction of a second to prevent excessive changes in H^+ concentration and pH. Although there are many buffer systems working within body fluids, four main systems exist.

- The bicarbonate/carbonic acid-buffer system
- The phosphate-buffer system
- The protein-buffer system
- The hemoglobin-buffer system.

The bicarbonate/carbonic acid buffer system is the major buffer system for fixed acids in the blood. (It buffers ~ 0.7 (70%) of the fixed acids in the plasma and ~ 0.3 (30%) of the fixed acids in the RBCs.) It is quantitatively the largest buffer system in the body, and is therefore the most important overall in regulating pH. Part of its importance derives from the fact that each of the components of this buffer system can be regulated via the lungs and kidneys:

- Carbonic acid (H_2CO_3) can be retained or exhaled as carbon dioxide (CO_2).
- Bicarbonate (HCO_3) can be retained or excreted by the kidney tubules as required by the body.

In the blood, the normal ratio of bicarbonate/carbonic acid is 20/1, so this system is heavily weighted toward buffering against excess acid production. Both components of this important buffer system can be regulated via the lungs and the kidneys. The weak acid component, carbonic acid (H_2CO_3), can be retained or exhaled as CO_2 via the lungs, while the salt component, bicarbonate (HCO_3) can be retained or excreted by the kidney tubules according to the body's needs.

The Respiratory (Lungs) Buffer Response

A normal by-product of cellular metabolism is CO_2. Carbon dioxide is carried in the blood to the lungs, where excess CO_2 combines with water (H_2O) to form carbonic acid (H_2CO_3) (Figure 2-2). The blood pH will change according to the level of carbonic acid present. This triggers the lungs to either increase or decrease the rate and depth of ventilation until the appropriate amount of

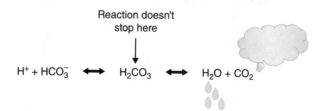

$$H^+ + HCO_3^- \longleftrightarrow H_2CO_3 \longleftrightarrow H_2O + CO_2$$

Reaction doesn't stop here

Figure 2-2 • The buffer response.

CO_2 has been reestablished. Activation of the lungs to compensate for an imbalance starts to occur within 1 to 3 minutes.

The Renal (Metabolic) Buffer Response

In an effort to maintain the pH of the blood within its normal range, the kidneys excrete or retain bicarbonate (HCO_3^-). As the blood pH decreases, the kidneys will compensate by retaining HCO_3^- and as the pH rises, the kidneys excrete HCO_3^- through the urine. Although the kidneys provide an excellent means of regulating acid-base balance, the system may take from hours to days to correct the imbalance. When the respiratory and renal systems are working together, they are able to keep the blood pH balanced by maintaining 1 part acid to 20 parts base.

Acid-Base Disorders

Respiratory Acidosis

Respiratory acidosis is defined as a pH less than 7.35 with a $PaCO_2$ greater than 45 mm Hg.

Acidosis is caused by an accumulation of CO_2 which combines with water in the body to produce carbonic acid, thus, lowering the pH of the blood. Any condition that results in hypoventilation can cause respiratory acidosis (see Figure 2-3). These conditions include:

- Central nervous system (CNS) depression related to head injury

- CNS depression related to medications such as narcotics, sedatives, or anesthesia

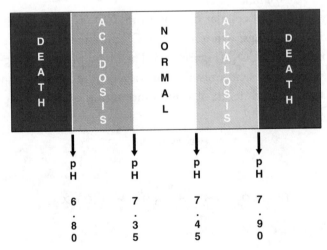

Figure 2-3 • pH extremes.

- Impaired respiratory muscle function related to spinal cord injury, neuro-muscular diseases, or neuromuscular blocking drugs
- Pulmonary disorders such as atelectasis, pneumonia, pneumothorax, pulmonary edema, or bronchial obstruction
- Massive pulmonary embolus
- Hypoventilation due to pain, chest wall injury/deformity, or abdominal distension

Increasing ventilation will correct respiratory acidosis. The method for achieving this will vary with the cause of hypoventilation. If the patient is unstable, manual ventilation with a bag-mask is indicated until the underlying problem can be addressed. After stabilization, rapidly resolvable causes are addressed immediately. Causes that can be treated rapidly include pneumothorax, pain, and CNS depression related to medications. If the cause cannot be readily resolved, the patient may require mechanical ventilation while treatment is rendered. Although patients with hypoventilation often require supplemental oxygen, it is important to remember that oxygen alone will not correct the problem.

What Went Wrong?

Signs and Symptoms of Respiratory Acidosis

Signs and symptoms depend on the rate and degree of PCO_2 because CO_2 rapidly diffuses across the blood-brain barrier. Signs and symptoms are a result of high CNS CO_2 concentrations (low CNS pH) and any accompanying hypoxemia.

Acute (or acutely worsening chronic) respiratory acidosis causes headache, confusion, anxiety, drowsiness, and stupor (CO_2 narcosis). Slowly developing, stable respiratory acidosis (as in COPD) may be well tolerated, but patients may have memory loss, sleep disturbances, excessive daytime sleepiness, and personality changes. Signs include gait disturbance, tremor, blunted deep tendon reflexes, myoclonic jerks, asterixis, and papilledema.

Respiratory Alkalosis

Respiratory alkalosis is defined as a pH greater than 7.45 with a $PaCO_2$ less than 35 mm Hg.

Any condition that causes hyperventilation can result in respiratory alkalosis. These conditions include:

- Psychological responses, such as anxiety or fear
- Pain

- Increased metabolic demands, such as fever, sepsis, pregnancy, or thyrotoxicosis
- Medications, such as respiratory stimulants
- Central nervous system lesions

What Went Wrong?

Signs and Symptoms of Respiratory Alkalosis

Signs and symptoms depend on the rate and degree of fall in PCO_2. Acute respiratory alkalosis causes light-headedness, confusion, peripheral and circumoral paresthesias, cramps, and syncope. Mechanism is thought to be from a change in cerebral blood flow and pH. Tachypnea or hyperpnea is often the only sign; carpopedal spasm may occur in severe cases. Chronic respiratory alkalosis is usually asymptomatic and has no distinctive signs.

Metabolic Acidosis

Metabolic acidosis is defined as a bicarbonate level less than 22 mEq/L with a pH of less than 7.35. Metabolic acidosis is caused by either a deficit of base in the bloodstream or an excess of acids, other than CO_2. Diarrhea and intestinal fistulas may cause decreased levels of base. Causes of increased acids include:

- Renal failure
- Diabetic ketoacidosis
- Anaerobic metabolism
- Starvation
- Salicylate intoxication

What Went Wrong?

Signs and Symptoms of Metabolic Acidosis

Mild acidemia is itself asymptomatic. More severe acidemia (pH < 7.10) may cause nausea, vomiting, and malaise. Symptoms may appear at higher pH if acidosis develops rapidly. The most characteristic sign is hyperpnea (long, deep breaths at a normal rate), reflecting a compensatory increase in alveolar ventilation.

Severe, acute acidemia predisposes to cardiac dysfunction with hypotension and shock, ventricular arrhythmias, and coma. Chronic acidemia causes bone demineralization disorders (ie, rickets, osteomalacia, and osteopenia).

As with most acid-base imbalances, the treatment of metabolic acidosis is dependent upon the cause. The presence of metabolic acidosis should spur a search for hypoxic tissue somewhere in the body. Hypoxemia can lead to anaerobic metabolism system-wide, but hypoxia of any tissue bed will produce metabolic acids as a result of anaerobic metabolism even if the PaO_2 is normal. The only appropriate way to treat this source of acidosis is to restore tissue perfusion to the hypoxic tissues. Other causes of metabolic acidosis should be considered after the possibility of tissue hypoxia has been addressed.

Metabolic Alkalosis

Metabolic alkalosis is defined as a bicarbonate level greater than 26 mEq/L and a pH greater than 7.45. Either an excess of base or a loss of acid within the body can cause metabolic alkalosis. Excess base occurs from ingestion of antacids, excess use of bicarbonate, or use of lactate in dialysis. Loss of acids may occur secondary to protracted vomiting, gastric suction, hypochloremia, excess administration of diuretics, or high levels of aldosterone. Metabolic alkalosis is one of the most difficult acid-base imbalances to treat. Bicarbonate excretion through the kidneys can be stimulated with drugs such as acetazolamide, but resolution of the imbalance will be slow. In severe cases, intravenous (IV) administration of acids maybe used.

What Went Wrong?

Signs and Symptoms of Metabolic Alkalosis

Signs and symptoms of mild alkalemia are usually related to the underlying disorder. More severe alkalemia increases protein binding of ionized ca^{++}, leading to hypocalcemia and subsequent headache, lethargy, and neuromuscular excitability, sometimes with delirium, tetany, and seizures. Alkalemia also lowers threshold for anginal symptoms and arrhythmias. Concomitant hypokalemia may cause weakness.

Components of the Arterial Blood Gas

The ABG provides the following values:

- **pH**: Measurement of acidity or alkalinity, based on the hydrogen ions (H^+) present.
- The normal range is 7.35 to 7.45.

KEY POINTS

pH>7.45 = alkalosis

pH<7.35 = acidosis

PO_2: The partial pressure of oxygen that is dissolved in arterial blood. The normal range is 80 to 100 mm Hg.

SaO_2: The arterial oxygen saturation. The normal range is 95% to 100%.

PCO_2: The amount of CO_2 dissolved in arterial blood. The normal range is 35 to 45 mm Hg.

KEY POINTS

PCO_2>45 mm Hg = acidosis

PCO_2<35 mm Hg = alkalosis

HCO_3: The calculated value of the amount of bicarbonate in the bloodstream. The normal range is 22 to 26 mEq/L.

KEY POINTS

HCO_3>26 mEq/L = alkalosis

HCO_3<22 mEq/L = acidosis

Base Excess (B.E.)

The base excess indicates the amount of excess or insufficient level of bicarbonate in the system. The normal range is −2 to +2 mEq/L

KEY POINT

A negative base excess indicates a base deficit in the blood.

Steps to an Arterial Blood Gas Interpretation

The ABG is used to evaluate both acid-base balance and oxygenation, each representing separate conditions. Acid-base evaluation requires a focus on three of the reported components: pH, $PaCO_2$, and HCO_3.

This process involves two basic steps.

Step One

Identify whether the levels of pH, PCO_2, and HCO_3 are abnormal. For each component, label it as "normal," "acidic," or "alkaline."

TABLE 2–2			
pH	7.30	(7.35-7.45)	ACID
PCO_2	55	(35-45)	ACID
HCO_3	26	(22-26)	NORMAL

The two matching values determine what the problem is (Table 2-2). In this case, an **ACIDOSIS!**

Step Two

If the ABG results are abnormal, determine if the abnormality is due to the kidneys (metabolic) or the lungs (respiratory) (Table 2-3).

TABLE 2–3				
pH	7.30	(7.35-7.45)	ACID	
PCO_2	55	(35-45)	ACID	= Lungs
HCO_3	26	(22-26)	NORMAL	= Kidneys

Match the two abnormalities.

Respiratory (lung problem) + Acidosis = Respiratory acidosis

Blood Gas Scenario One

You are treating a 55-year-old man who has been treated for recurring bowel obstruction. He has been experiencing intractable vomiting for the past several hours despite the use of antiemetics. His ABG result is as follows:

pH 7.50
PCO_2 42 mm Hg
HCO_3 33 mEq/L

Step One

Identify whether the levels of pH, PCO_2, and HCO_3 are abnormal (Table 2-4). For each component, label it as "normal," "acid," or "alkaline."

TABLE 2–4			
pH	7.50	(7.35-7.45)	ALKALINE
PCO$_2$	42	(35-45)	NORMAL
HCO$_3$	33	(22-26)	ALKALINE

The two matching values determine what the problem is. In this case, an ALKALOSIS.

Step Two

If the ABG results are abnormal, determine if the abnormality is due to the kidneys (metabolic) or the lungs (respiratory) (Table 2-5).

TABLE 2–5				
pH	7.50	(7.35-7.45)	ALKALINE	
PaCO$_2$	42	(35-45)	NORMAL	= Lungs
HCO$_3$	33	(22-26)	ALKALINE	= Kidneys

Match the two abnormalities.

Kidneys (metabolic) + Alkalosis = Metabolic alkalosis

Blood Gas Scenario Two

You are treating a 55-year-old woman who is exhibiting signs of sepsis. Here is her ABG result:

pH 7.31
PCO$_2$ 39 mm Hg
HCO$_3$ 17 mEq/L

Step One

Identify whether the levels of pH, PCO$_2$, and HCO$_3$ are abnormal (Table 2-6). For each component, label it as "normal," "acid," or "alkaline."

TABLE 2–6			
pH	7.31	(7.35-7.45)	ACIDOSIS
PaCO$_2$	39	(35-45)	NORMAL
HCO$_3$	17	(22-26)	ACIDOSIS

The two matching values determine what the problem is. In this case, an ACIDOSIS.

Step Two

If the ABG results are abnormal, determine if the abnormality is due to the kidneys (metabolic)or the lungs (respiratory) (Table 2-7).

TABLE 2–7			
pH	7.31	(7.35-7.45)	ACIDOSIS
PaCO$_2$	39	(35-45)	NORMAL = Lungs
HCO$_3$	17	(22-26)	ACIDOSIS = Kidneys

Match the two abnormalities.

Kidneys (metabolic) + Acidosis = Metabolic acidosis

Blood Gas Scenario Three

You are treating a 34-year-old woman who is diagnosed with thyrotoxicosis. Her blood gas results are as follows:

pH 7.50
PCO$_2$ 30 mm Hg
HCO$_3$ 24mEq/L

Step One

Identify whether the levels of pH, PCO$_2$, and HCO$_3$ are abnormal (Table 2-8). For each component, label it as "Normal," "acid," or "alkaline."

TABLE 2–8			
pH	7.50	(7.35-7.45)	ALKALOSIS
PaCO$_2$	30	(35-45)	ALKALOSIS
HCO$_3$	24	(22-26)	NORMAL

The two matching values determine what the problem is. In this case, an ALKALOSIS.

Step Two

If the ABG results are abnormal, determine if the abnormality is due to the kidneys (metabolic)or the lungs (respiratory) (Table 2-9).

TABLE 2–9			
pH	7.50	(7.35-7.45)	ALKALOSIS
PaCO$_2$	30	(35-45)	ALKALOSIS = Lungs
HCO$_3$	24	(22-26)	NORMAL = Kidneys

Match the two abnormalities.

Respiratory (lung problem) + Alkalosis = Respiratory Alkalosis

Blood Gas Scenario Four

You are treating a 19-year-old female with head injury. Her blood gas results are as follows:

pH 7.38
PCO$_2$ 56 mm Hg
HCO$_3$ 35 mEq/L

Step One

Identify whether the levels of pH, pCO$_2$ and HCO$_3$ are abnormal (Table 2-10). For each component, label it as "Normal," "acid," or "alkaline."

TABLE 2–10			
pH	7.38	(7.35-7.45)	NORMAL
PaCO$_2$	56	(35-45)	ACIDOSIS
HCO$_3$	35	(22-26)	ALKALOSIS

Notice now, for the first time, that both the PCO$_2$ and the HCO$_3$ are abnormal. This indicates that there is some degree of compensation taking place. This will require a slightly different approach to the blood gas analysis.

Compensation

So far we have looked at simple ABG values without any evidence of compensation occurring. Now see what happens when an acid-base imbalance exists over a period of time.

When a patient develops an acid-base imbalance, the body attempts to compensate. Remember that the lungs and the kidneys are the primary buffer response systems in the body. The body tries to overcome either a respiratory or metabolic dysfunction in an attempt to return the pH into the normal range.

A patient can be uncompensated, partially compensated, or fully compensated. How do you know when compensation is occurring? When an acid-base disorder is either uncompensated or partially compensated, the pH remains outside the normal range. In fully compensated states, the pH has returned to within the normal range, although the other values may still be abnormal. Be aware that neither system has the ability to overcompensate. In our first three examples, the patients were uncompensated. In each case, the pH was outside of the normal range, the primary source of the acid-base imbalance was readily identified, but the third value (the compensatory buffering system) remained in the normal range. Let's return to our ABG results where there is evidence of compensation.

TABLE 2−11			
pH	7.38	(7.35-7.45)	NORMAL
PaCO$_2$	56	(35-45)	ACIDOSIS
HCO$_3$	35	(22-26)	ALKALOSIS

As you might recall, in step one, we determined that both the PCO$_2$ and HCO$_3$ were abnormal, indicating the presence of some degree of compensation. Now we need to know two things.

First, are we dealing with an acidosis or an alkalosis? Second, how do you know which system (respiratory or metabolic) is the primary problem and which is compensating? To determine this, we must go back and look at the pH in a slightly different manner.

Step Two

If both the PCO$_2$ and the HCO$_3$ are abnormal, but the pH is in the normal range, look at the pH again. Instead of using a "normal range" of 7.35-7.45 as we have been doing, we are going to use the single value of 7.40 as our only "normal." Any pH of < 7.40 is now going to be considered **acidosis**. If pH > 7.40 it is now going to be considered alkalosis. Look at our pH in this example. The pH is < 7.40 (Table 2-12).

TABLE 2−12			
pH	7.38	(7.40)	ACIDOSIS
PaCO$_2$	56	(35-45)	ACIDOSIS
HCO$_3$	35	(22-26)	ALKALOSIS

The two matching values determine what the problem is. In this case, an ACIDOSIS.

What Went Wrong?

We only use a single value of 7.40 as "normal" when both PCO_2 and HCO_3 are abnormal and the original pH is normal.

Step Three

Now, for the two matching values, determine if the abnormality is due to the kidneys (metabolic) or the lungs (respiratory) (Table 2-13).

TABLE 2–13			
pH	7.38	(7.40)	ACIDOSIS
PaCO$_2$	56	(35-45)	ACIDOSIS = Lungs
HCO$_3$	35	(22-26)	ALKALOSIS

Match the two abnormalities.

Respiratory (lungs) + Acidosis = Respiratory Acidosis

Finally, we need to determine if the condition is partially or completely compensated.

Blood Gas Scenario Five

Jane Doe is admitted to the ICU. Her admission laboratory work reveals an ABG with the following values:

pH 7.45
PCO_2 48 mm Hg
HCO_3 28 mEq/L

Step One

Identify whether the levels of pH, PCO_2 and HCO_3 are abnormal (Table 2-14). For each component, label it as "Normal," "acid," or "alkaline."

TABLE 2–14			
pH	7.45	(7.35-7.45)	NORMAL
PCO$_2$	48	(35-45)	ACIDOSIS
HCO$_3$	28	(22-26)	ALKALOSIS

Because both the PCO_2 and HCO_3 are abnormal, we know that some degree of compensation is occurring!

Step Two

Because the initial pH is normal, we must look again at the pH using 7.40 as the single value for "normal." Label the pH as acidotic or alkalotic (Table 2-15).

TABLE 2–15			
pH	7.45	(7.40)	ALKALOSIS
PCO$_2$	48	(35-45)	ACIDOSIS
HCO$_3$	28	(22-26)	ALKALOSIS

The two matching values determine what the problem is. In this case, an ALKALOSIS.

Step Three

For the two matching values, determine if the abnormality is due to the kidneys (metabolic) or the lungs (respiratory) (Table 2-16).

TABLE 2–16			
pH	7.45	(7.40)	ALKALOSIS
PCO$_2$	48	(35-45)	ACIDOSIS
HCO$_3$	28	(22-26)	ALKALOSIS = Kidneys

Match the two abnormalities.

Kidneys (metabolic) + Alkalosis = Metabolic alkalosis

Finally, we need to determine if the condition is partially or completely compensated. In this example, because the pH is 7.45 (within the range of 7.35-7.45), the condition is fully compensated. Our final ABG analysis indicates that we have a compensated metabolic alkalosis.

Blood Gas Scenario Six

You are treating a trauma patient with an altered mental status. His initial ABG result is as follows:

pH 7.33
PCO$_2$ 62 mm Hg
HCO$_3$ 35 mEq/L

Step One

Identify whether the pH, PCO$_2$ and HCO$_3$ are abnormal (Table 2-17). For each component, label it as "normal," "acid," or "alkaline."

TABLE 2–17			
pH	7.33	(7.35-7.45)	ACIDOSIS
PCO$_2$	62	(35-45)	ACIDOSIS
HCO$_3$	35	(22-26)	ALKALOSIS

Because both the PCO$_2$ and HCO$_3$ are abnormal, we know that some degree of compensation is occurring.

Step Two

Because the PCO$_2$ and HCO$_3$ are both abnormal, it indicates that some degree of compensation is occurring. However, because the pH is also abnormal, we do not need to look at it again since it is already labeled as abnormal (Table 2-18).

TABLE 2–18			
pH	7.33	(7.35-7.45)	ACIDOSIS
PCO$_2$	62	(35-45)	ACIDOSIS
HCO$_3$	35	(22-26)	ALKALOSIS

The two matching values determine what the problem is. In this case, an ACIDOSIS.

Step Three

For the two matching values, determine if the abnormality is due to the kidneys (metabolic) or the lungs (respiratory) (Table 2-19).

TABLE 2–19			
pH	7.33	(7.35-7.45)	ACIDOSIS
PCO$_2$	62	(35-45)	ACIDOSIS = Lungs
HCO$_3$	35	(22-26)	ALKALOSIS

Match the two abnormalities.

Respiratory (lungs) + Acidosis = Respiratory acidosis

Finally, we need to determine if the condition is partially or completely compensated.

In this example, because the pH is 7.33 (outside the range of 7.35-7.45), the condition is only partially compensated. Our final ABG analysis indicates that we have a partially compensated respiratory acidosis.

Blood Gas Scenario Seven

A 54-year-old woman is admitted to Emergency Department (ED). Here are the last ABG results:

pH 7.29
PCO₂ 30 mm Hg
HCO₃ 18 mEq/L

Step One

Identify whether the pH, PCO_2, and HCO_3 are abnormal. For each component, label it as "normal," "acid," or "alkaline" (Table 2-20).

TABLE 2−20			
pH	7.29	(7.35-7.45)	ACIDOSIS
PCO₂	30	(35-45)	ALKALOSIS
HCO₃	18	(22-26)	ACIDOSIS

Because both the PCO_2 and HCO_3 are abnormal, we know that some degree of compensation is occurring.

Step Two

Here, the pH is out of the normal range and we have already labeled it as acidosis (Table 2-21).

TABLE 2−21			
pH	7.29	(7.35-7.45)	ACIDOSIS
PCO₂	30	(35-45)	ALKALOSIS
HCO₃	18	(22-26)	ACIDOSIS

The two matching values determine what the problem is. In this case, an ACIDOSIS.

Step Three

For the two matching values, determine if the abnormality is due to the kidneys (metabolic) or the lungs (respiratory) (Table 2-22).

TABLE 2−22			
pH	7.29	(7.35-7.45)	ACIDOSIS
PCO₂	30	(35-45)	ALKALOSIS
HCO₃	18	(22-26)	ACIDOSIS = Kidneys

Match the two abnormalities.

Metabolic (kidneys) + Acidosis = Metabolic acidosis

Finally, we need to determine if the condition is partially or completely compensated.

In this example, because the pH is 7.29 (outside the range of 7.35-7.45), the condition is only partially compensated. Our final ABG analysis indicates that we have a partially compensated metabolic acidosis.

KEY POINT

Although the focus of this chapter has been on interpretation of acid-base imbalances, the ABG can also be used to evaluate blood oxygenation. The component of the ABG used to evaluate this is the PaO_2. Remember that the normal blood PaO_2 value is 80-100 mm Hg.

Oxyhemoglobin Dissociation Curve

Figure 2-4 depicts one of nature's most complicated and unique creations, a protein molecule called hemoglobin. Each hemoglobin molecule is made up of 10,000 atoms, 4 of which are iron atoms that act as magnets to attract and hold the oxygen molecules. Each iron atom rests on a heme platform which serves to release the oxygen, out in the peripheral tissues. Each red blood cell (RBC) contains about 250 million molecules of hemoglobin, each cc of blood contains 5 billion RBCs. You have approximately 5,000 cc's of blood in your

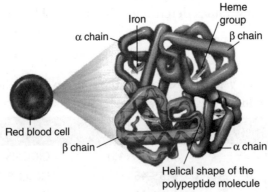

Figure 2-4 • Hemoglobin molecule.
Mader, Sylvia S. *Inquiry into Life*, 8th ed., ISBN 13: 9780697251817.

vascular system. The reason we have so much hemoglobin is because oxygen does not easily dissolve in water (about 3% of all our oxygen is in the serum—the rest is bound to hemoglobin), so we have developed this unique system of oxygen transportation to meet our needs. When oxygen is bound to hemoglobin, it is called oxyhemoglobin.

The air around us comprises many substances. The major gasses are: nitrogen, oxygen, CO_2, and water vapor. The minor gasses (accounting for less than 1%) are argon, xenon, ozone, carbon monoxide, nitrous oxide, helium, and so on. Other substances float around in this "sea" of gasses such as organic and inorganic dusts and vapors.

The principal or most abundant gas is nitrogen (N_2) accounting for 78% of the molecules in an air sample. Nitrogen is a colorless, odorless, inert gas. This means that it does not easily react with other chemicals. This does not mean that nitrogen is unnecessary to us. We do absorb nitrogen from the air, and it is necessary for normal life functions. At the alveolar membrane, nitrogen molecules are constantly moving into and out of our blood. There is an equilibrium reached between our body and the nitrogen in the atmosphere. You can, however, go short periods without breathing nitrogen. When you give your patient 100% oxygen, the patient is deprived of the nitrogen in room air. Gradually, your body exhales the nitrogen present in the cells and bloodstream. Remember your lessons on diffusion? If the alveolus is filled with 100% oxygen, then the nitrogen in the blood moves from the area of higher concentration to an area of lower concentration. Because the airway is being flushed with pure oxygen, there is a large gradient between the capillary bed and alveolus. A large amount of nitrogen can be removed in a short time.

If a patient were to receive pure oxygen for days, nearly all of the body's nitrogen gas would be removed. You have probably heard of oxygen toxicity, it is a misnomer because most of the damage occurs from the deficiency of nitrogen. Knowing these principles helps you understand other issues and treatments in medicine.

Example Patients with small, stable pneumothoraces (10-20% collapse) will be sent home by the ED. The pocket of air will gradually be absorbed in a weeks' time. Some physicians have the patient breath 100% oxygen for 30 minutes twice a day for 2 days. The air trapped in the pleural space is usually absorbed in only 24 hours.

Can you explain the mechanism?

Oxygen or O_2 is a colorless, odorless gas that is present in our atmosphere along with other gasses. Oxygen accounts for 20.9% (often rounded to 21) of the air around us. Oxygen is an essential component in the citric acid cycle. Oxygen is used by the cells in our body to produce the energy needed for heat production and cellular energy. Too much or too little oxygen can cause illness and death. This is why it has become necessary for health care professionals to be able to quantify the amount of oxygen in the bloodstream.

Years ago, the only method of determining the oxygen content of arterial blood was to puncture an artery with a needle and send that blood to a laboratory. The result came back as the "partial pressure" of oxygen dissolved in the total sample. This may be a new concept for some and we need to simplify the concept of measuring gasses that are dissolved in a liquid. At sea level, the atmosphere pushes down on us like the water would if you were on the bottom of the ocean. Even though you don't feel it, your body is being pressed by 14.696 lbs per square inch or 760 mm Hg. If you were in an atmosphere of pure oxygen, your arterial pressure of oxygen would nearly equal 760 mm Hg in the bloodstream. Because our atmosphere is only 20.9% oxygen, we need to find 20.9% of 760 mm Hg to determine how much oxygen (or the partial pressure) is being forced into our blood. 20.9% of 760 mm Hg is 158.8 after adjusting for airway dead space, elevation, patient temperature, and water vapor; a healthy patient breathing room air can have a PaO_2 that typically ranges from 90-106 Torr. The PaO_2 can go much higher than this if the patient is breathing supplemental oxygen and/or under increased barometric pressure such as a hyperbaric chamber.

The oxyhemoglobin dissociation curve is a tool used to show the relationship between oxygen saturation and the PaO_2. The strength with which oxygen binds to the hemoglobin molecule has important clinical implications. If the oxygen binds too loosely, the hemoglobin may give up its oxygen before it reaches the tissues in need. If the oxygen binds too tightly, it may not transfer to the tissues at all. The strength of the oxygen-hemoglobin bond is graphically represented by the oxyhemoglobin dissociation curve (Figure 2-5).

Several variables affect the affinity of the oxygen molecule to hemoglobin. Conditions that cause enhanced release of the oxygen molecule include acidosis, fever, elevated CO_2 levels, and increased 2,3-diphosphoglycerate (2,3-DPG, a by-product of glucose metabolism). This change in affinity is called a shift to the right. Conditions that keep the oxygen molecule tightly attached to hemoglobin include hypothermia, alkalosis, low PCO_2, and decrease in 2,3-DPG. This change is called a shift to the left. A shift to the left has more negative implications for the patient than a shift to the right.

If evaluation of blood oxygenation is required, you can assess this by adding one additional step to your ABG analysis.

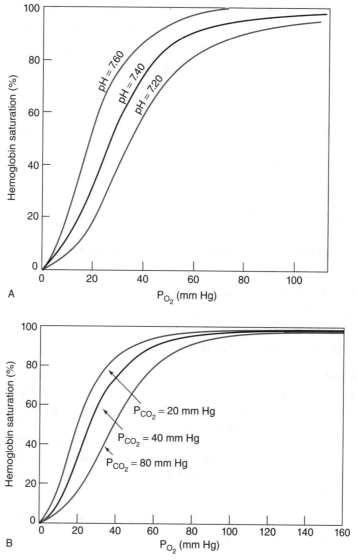

Figure 2-5 • Oxyhemoglobin dissociation curve.
Reproduced with permission from Levitzky MG, ed. *Pulmonary Physiology*. 7th ed. 2007. New York: Copyright © McGraw-Hill Education. All rights reserved.

Step Four

Assess the PaO_2. A value below 80 mm Hg can indicates hypoxemia, depending on the age of the patient. Correction of a patient's blood oxygenation level may be accomplished through a combination of augmenting the means of oxygen delivery and correcting existing conditions that are shifting the oxyhemoglobin curve.

Thus understanding ABGs can sometimes be confusing. A logical and systematic approach using these steps makes interpretation much easier. Applying the concepts of acid-base balance will help the healthcare provider follow the progress of a patient and evaluate the effectiveness of care being provided.

REVIEW QUESTIONS

Following are the ABG values:

pH 7.56
$PaCO_2$ 31 mm Hg
HCO_3 27 mEq/L
PaO_2 56 mm Hg

1. What is (are) the most likely acid-base state(s) in the patient?

   A. Acute respiratory alkalosis
   B. Chronic respiratory alkalosis
   C. Respiratory alkalosis and metabolic alkalosis
   D. Respiratory acidosis and metabolic acidosis
   E. Respiratory alkalosis and metabolic acidosis

Correct answer is c.

Explanation: The subject is hyperventilating with an elevated pH, indicating respiratory alkalosis. However, when hyperventilation bicarbonate goes down from the simple excretion of CO_2 in the hydration equation; $CO_2 + H_2O$ <----> $HCO_3^- + H^+$. As CO_2 is excreted both bicarbonate and H^+ fall. With simple hyperventilation and no other acid-base disorder the HCO_3^- should fall slightly from the normal value of 24 mEq/L, and be about 22 to 23 mEq/L. In this example it is 27 mEq/L, indicating a concomitant mild metabolic alkalosis.

2. Which of the following changes will most increase arterial oxygen delivery?

   A. PaO_2 from 60 to 95 mm Hg
   B. Cardiac output from 4 to 5 L/min
   C. Hemoglobin from 9 to 10 grams%
   D. Atmospheric pressure from 1 to 2 atmospheres
   E. Arterial pH from 7.30 to 7.50

Correct answer is c.

Explanation: Oxygen delivery is oxygen content x cardiac output.

- The change in PaO_2 will increase SaO_2 from about 90% to 98%, in effect increasing CaO_2 about 9% and O_2 delivery about the same.
- This is a 25% increase in cardiac output, which will increase oxygen delivery 25%.

- This is an 11% increase in oxygen content, which will increase O_2 delivery the same percentage, 11%.
- This change will increase PaO_2 from about 100 to 200 mm Hg, for a negligible increase in SaO_2 and oxygen content.
- This change will shift the O_2 dissociation curve to the left and increase SaO_2 slightly, perhaps by 2% to 3%.

Following are the ABG values:

pH 7.40
$PaCO_2$ 20 mm Hg
HCO_3 12 mEq/L

3. **What is (are) the most likely acid-base state(s) in the patient?**
    A. Metabolic acidosis with full compensation
    B. Respiratory alkalosis with full compensation
    C. Metabolic acidosis and respiratory alkalosis
    D. Metabolic acidosis and metabolic alkalosis
    E. Normal acid-base state

Correct answer is c.

4. **A normal pH with abnormal $PaCO_2$ or HCO_3 indicates two or more acid-base disorders. Full compensation (back to baseline) is never achieved with a single acid-base disorder. All of the following are true about non-arterial assessment of oxygenation and acid-base balance except:**

    A. if venous CO_2 (measured as part of standard electrolyte panel) is truly abnormal, the patient has some type of acid-base disorder.
    B. in a hemodynamically stable patient, venous blood gases measured from central venous blood can be used to assess acid-base status.
    C. if venous blood can be used in lieu of arterial blood to measure blood carboxy-hemoglobin.
    D. if the bicarbonate gap, which is ($Na^+ - Cl^- - 39$), can diagnose a metabolic alkalosis even when there is increased anion gap.
    E. in a stable patient with normal lungs, the difference between $PaCO_2$ and end-tidal PCO_2 is 10 to 15 mm Hg.

Correct answer is e.

Explanation: In a normal person end-tidal PCO_2 is equal to $PaCO_2$. All other statements are true.

A patient presents with the following ABGs, drawn on room air ($FIO_2 = 0.21$).

pH 7.40
PCO_2 40 mm Hg
PO_2 82 mm Hg
HCO_3 24 mEq/L

5. **Which of the following statements is most accurate?**

    A. The patient does not have an acid-base disorder.

    B. To determine if there is an acid-base disorder you need to know the measured serum bicarbonate, since the HCO_3 from blood gases is only a calculation.

    C. Need to know patient's respiratory rate, as $PaCO_2$ may be inappropriately "normal" and signify a respiratory acidosis.

    D. A patient can have normal blood gases if two metabolic acid-base disorders oppose to give normal bicarbonate.

    E. The PaO_2 is lower than predicted for a patient breathing room air.

Correct answer is d.
Explanation: Metabolic acidosis and metabolic alkalosis can coexist, so the patient ends up with a normal HCO_3 and $PaCO_2$. Serum electrolytes can make the diagnosis by showing increased anion gap; in the presence of normal HCO_3, increased AG would indicate the two disorders.

A patient with respiratory failure has the following ABGs ($FIO_2 = 0.21$, sea level):

pH 7.20
PCO_2 70 mm Hg
PO_2 60 mm Hg
SaO_2 86%

6. **Which of the following is the least likely cause of these abnormal blood gases?**

    A. Congestive heart failure

    B. Narcotic overdose

    C. Myasthenia gravis

    D. Flail chest

    E. Guillain Barré syndrome

Correct answer is c.
Explanation: All of these conditions can lead to respiratory acidosis, but congestive heart failure would be least likely to do so without increasing the A-a O_2 difference. Alveolar PO_2 in this example is $0.21(760 - 43) - 1.2(PaCO_2) = 150 - 84 = 66$. Thus the $(PAO_2 - PaO_2)$, or so-called "A-a gradient" is normal at about 6 mm Hg. Since the other conditions can cause respiratory acidosis without involving the lung parenchyma, and thus without raising $(PAO_2 - PaO_2)$, CHF is the correct answer.

A 30-year-old man, previously healthy, is complaining of dyspnea after suffering smoke inhalation. Measured carboxyhemoglobin is 20% and hemoglobin content = 15%. He has the following blood gas values:

PaO_2 80 mm Hg (on room air at sea level)
$PaCO_2$ 32 mm Hg
pH 7.34
SaO_2 96% (calculated)

7. **Examination shows clear lungs to auscultation. From this information alone, you can determine that:**

    A. his actual SaO_2 is much lower than the calculated value.
    B. there is no lung abnormality present, though pulmonary disease could develop in the ensuing 24 hours.
    C. he has a mild metabolic acidosis associated with an increased anion gap.
    D. his arterial oxygen content is in the normal range.
    E. None of the above.

Correct answer is a.
Explanation: Given 20% carboxyhemoglobin, his actual SaO_2 (which is the % of hemoglobin bound to oxygen) cannot be more than 80%. As to: (b), a lung abnormality could be present, especially since his (PAO_2—PaO_2) is somewhat increased; (c) no electrolyte information is given, so you don't know if he has an increased anion gap; (d) no hemoglobin content is given, so you don't know his oxygen content; (e) is incorrect, since (a) is the answer.

8. **All of the following are true about cyanosis except that:**

    A. for cyanosis to manifest there needs to be 5% of deoxygenated hemoglobin in the capillaries.
    B. patients with normal hemoglobin manifest cyanosis at higher SaO_2 values than patients with anemia.
    C. cyanosis can be caused by excess methemoglobin, which is $HbFe^{+3}$.
    D. for methemoglobin to cause cyanosis, the PaO_2 generally has to be <80 mm Hg.
    E. some drugs may cause cyanosis without causing vasoconstriction, or any impairment in PaO_2, SaO_2, or oxygen content.

Correct answer is d.
Explanation: Methemoglobin can cause cyanosis with a normal PaO_2. All the other statements are true.

9. **A 40-year-old patient is admitted to the ICU with the following laboratory values:**

BLOOD GASES

pH 7.40
PCO_2 38 mm Hg
HCO_3 24 mEq/L
PO_2 88 mm Hg (on room air)

ELECTROLYTES, BUN AND CREATININE

Na 149 mEq/L
K 3.8 mEq/L
Cl 100 mEq/L
CO_2 24 mEq/L
BUN 110 mg%
Creatinine 8.7 mg%

Which statement best describes the disorder(s)?
    A. Normal electrolytes, normal blood gases
    B. Abnormal electrolytes and abnormal blood gases
    C. Metabolic acidosis
    D. Metabolic alkalosis
    E. Metabolic acidosis and metabolic alkalosis

Correct answer is e.
Explanation: Electrolytes are not normal, since the anion gap is increased: AG = 149 − (100 + 24) = 25. Thus, there is at least a metabolic acidosis. Furthermore, since CO_2 is "normal" at 24, despite an increased anion gap, there must aso be a metabolic alkalosis.

10. **Below are two sets of blood gases:**
Patient A: pH 7.48, $PaCO_2$ 34 mm Hg, PaO_2 85 mm Hg, SaO_2 95%, Hemoglobin 7%
Patient B: pH 7.32, $PaCO_2$ 74 mm Hg, PaO_2 55 mm Hg, SaO_2 85%, Hemoglobin 15%

Which is the most correct statement?
    A. B is more hypoxemic because PaO_2 is lower than A.
    B. B is more hypoxemic because SaO_2 is lower than A.
    C. A is more hypoxemic because A-a gradient is higher than B.
    D. A is more hypoxemic because O_2 content is lower than B.
    E. The differences balance out and neither A nor B is more hypoxemic than the other.

Correct answer is d.
Explanation: Hypoxemia means low oxygen content in the blood. If you don't have oxygen content, then you might use PaO_2 and/or SaO_2 as a surrogate for assessing hypoxemia, but here you do have oxygen content information. The oxygen contents are (excluding contribution of dissolved O_2):
Patient A: $1.34 \times 7 \times 0.95 = 8.91$ mL O_2/dL
Patient B: $1.34 \times 15 \times 0.85 = 17.09$ mL O_2/dL
Clearly, patient A is more hypoxemic despite having a higher PaO_2 and SaO_2 than patient B.

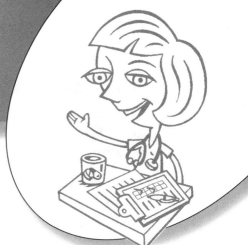

chapter 3

Pathophysiology of Apnea and Hypoxia

At the end of this chapter, you will be able to:

1 Define and distinguish between hypoxia, hypoxemia, anoxia, and asphyxia.

2 Describe the clinical significance in distinguishing between the common causes of hypoxia.

3 Describe clinically important causes of arterial hypoxemia.

KEY TERMS

Anemic (hypemic) hypoxia
Diffusion impairment
Histotoxic hypoxia
Hypoventilation
Hypoxia

Hypoxic hypoxia
Low inspired oxygen
Right to left shunt
Stagnant hypoxia
Ventilation-perfusion dissimilarity

Often times in emergency medical services (EMS), emergency medical technicians (EMTs) and paramedics are asked to respond, evaluate, and transport patients with hypoxemia. The fact that patients are visibly short of breath may all be initial reasons why EMS is called. Before delving into a differential diagnosis, it is essential to rule out life-threatening conditions, take a good history, look at key features of the physical examination, know what tests are helpful, and then understand some of the mechanisms of hypoxia. A patient with hypoxia may show impaired judgment, mental confusion, and motor incoordination. As it progresses, patients may become fatigued, drowsy, and inattentive, and have delayed reaction time. Finally, hypoxia can affect the brainstem centers and cause death.

What is hypoxia?

Between oxygen (O_2) requirements of cells and the actual oxygen supply can arise differences due to disturbance of some processes. The result is the lack of oxygen in tissues. It means that oxygenation is not effective. In this situation a condition develops which is called hypoxia.

Hypoxia as a term is used frequently. But it should be used exclusively in relation to the condition in which the oxygenation at the cellular level is impaired or inadequate. The partial pressure of oxygen (pO_2) in tissue is usually lower. It can be the consequence of disturbed oxygenation. Under the condition of hypoxia, oxidative phosphorylation is disturbed, and therefore, the generation of energy in the cell is impaired. During the lack of O_2, the ATP to adenosine diphosphate (ADP) ratio falls ten-fold. Glycolysis is a series of chemical reactions, by which glucose is converted to pyruvate and hydrogen (which does not need O_2). Glycolysis can function during hypoxia; the net gain of ATP however, is low. If the supply of O_2 is normal, glycolysis cannot continue, because it is inhibited by the feedback mechanism of pyruvate and hydrogen. Under anaerobic conditions pyruvate and hydrogen are converted to lactate, which inhibits the glycolysis by the feedback mechanism. Anaerobic glycolysis provides energy during the insufficient O_2 supply. This way of energy gaining cannot be useful for a long period of time. After a certain time it leads to the impairment of cells. A higher level of lactic acid during hypoxia shifts the pH in the cell to acid values. When the lactic acid diffuses from the cells into the environment, metabolic acidosis develops very quickly. In this situation the efficiency of the Na^+/K^+ pump decreases, as there is not enough energy for its activity. Finally, the low efficiency of the Na^+/K^+ pump results in an accumulation of Na^+ in the cells and the escape of K^+ into the intercellular space.

The changes in ion concentrations are the underlying cause of osmotic edema of mitochondria and cells. These changes affect just the metabolically active cells. The function of mitochondria could recover by an adequate O_2 supply, but if the pH drops without control, intracellular enzymes can be released damaging the intracellular structures including the nucleus. This will inhibit the chemical reactions and the homeostatic control of cells. These changes ultimately result in cellular death. The effect of hypoxia is identical in all types of cells. First, anaerobic metabolic processes take place, subsequently lactic acid is produced.

Mitochondrial

ATP production decreases, which causes the pH to shift to an acid value. Finally, acidosis in cells and irreversible changes in cellular structure and their nuclei due to the released intracellular enzymes develop.

Causes of Hypoxia

The term hypoxia can be generally defined as a state of O_2 deficiency or lack of oxygen. This reduced or insufficient O_2 supply to the tissues can cause impairment of bodily functions which may become irreversible if allowed to go untreated.

There are four types of hypoxia, each of these having a number of possible causes:

1. Hypoxic hypoxia
2. Anemic (hypemic) hypoxia
3. Stagnant hypoxia
4. Histotoxic hypoxia

A patient with O_2 deficiency may be suffering from a single cause or any combination of causes from one or more types of hypoxia.

- **Hypoxic Hypoxia**: Breathing air or a gas which contains a lower than normal PO_2 (ie, high altitudes, rebreathing in a closed space)
  - decrease in pulmonary ventilation (ie, pneumothorax, partial airway obstruction, and drug-induced respiratory depression)
  - abnormal lung function (ie, asthma, fibrotic disease, fluid filled alveoli as with pulmonary edema, pneumonia, hemorrhage, or drowning)
  - arterio-venous shunting (ie, some congenital heart defects allow for mixing of arterial and venous blood)
- **Anemic Hypoxia**: Reduced or altered hemoglobin (Hb). In this case, blood does not have a normal O_2 carrying capacity. There is either a reduced concentration of Hb (anemia) or the Hb that is there, has a reduced ability to chemically unite with oxygen. Some common causes are:
  - any type of anemia causing a reduction in Hb concentration
  - certain poisonings which chemically alter Hb
  - Hb combined with a gas other than O_2, ie, carbon monoxide

What Went Wrong?

Cyanosis, due to the color of deoxygenated blood, may be present in either type of hypoxia. It should be noted that cyanosis may be absent or reduced in the

TABLE 3–1 Blood Gas Disorders					
	Arterial Blood		**Venous Blood**		**Does supplemental oxygen increase PaO_2 substantially?**
	PO_2	PCO_2	PO_2	PCO_2	
Hypoxemia					
Hypoventilation	↓	↑	↓	↑	Yes
↓P_1O_2	↓	↓	↓	↓	Yes
R–L shunt	↓	Normal	↓	Normal	No
Diffusion defect	↓	Normal	↓	Normal	Yes
VA/Q inequality	↓	Normal	↓	Normal	Yes
Tissue hypoxia					
Anemic hypoxia	Normal	Normal	↓	Normal	No
CO poisoning	Normal	Normal	↓	Normal	Possibly
Stagnant hypoxia	Normal	Normal	↓	Normal	No
Histotoxic hypoxia	Normal	Normal	↑	Normal	No

anemic patient, or the patient poisoned with carbon monoxide. When carboxy hemoglobin is greater than 20% "cherry red skin" originally described in EMS textbooks is rarely seen on live patients. In fact, it is typically seen on postmortem.

- **Stagnant Hypoxia**: Any shock state in which there is widespread inadequate tissue perfusion, hence inadequate tissue oxygenation. This form of hypoxia refers to end-organ perfusion. With this type of hypoxia, both the O_2 carrying capacity and the PO_2 maybe normal. What causes this problem is an extreme blood flow deficit. This serious lack of blood flow may be localized to a specific region or may be generalized throughout the body. Some of the major causes are:
  - general—hypovolemic shock, cardiogenic shock
  - localized—thrombosis, embolus, vasoconstriction
- **Histotoxic Hypoxia**: While the blood's ability to pick up and transport O_2 may remain unaffected, a problem may also exist at the cellular level. An action by a toxic substance may prevent the diffusion of O_2 into the cells or may prevent the cells from utilizing oxygen. Cyanide is a poison which will cause this type of hypoxia.

Physical Findings Associated with Tissue Hypoxia

1. CNS impairment: Restlessness, confusion, unsteady gait, slurred speech, stupor, and coma
2. Tachycardia (early): Ventricular dysrhythmias and bradycardia (late)
3. Tachypnea, diaphoresis, pallor with or without cyanosis

Hypoxia of tissues can arise when the oxygen demand of cells is very high. This causes the metabolic activity to rise. Disorders of ventilation and of exchange of gases cause a decreased saturation of arterial blood with oxygen. This is why hypoxic hypoxia occurs.

Disorders of perfusion can cause the capacity of blood for oxygen transfer to be poorly utilized. Certain toxic substances can inhibit the transport of electrons in the respiratory chain, which in turn can cause oxidative phosphorylation to decrease or stop. This kind of hypoxia (histotoxic hypoxia) is caused by cyanide and arsenic compounds. In some diseases the oxygen supply is normal, yet it fails to satisfy the enormously increased demands. This occurs when the metabolic processes increase markedly. Increased demands for oxygen supply occur during physical effort, fever, anxiety, and stress. In severe injury, burns, and sepsis, the body is permanently on the border of tissue hypoxia. Increased oxygen supply demands may also be caused by hyperthyroidism. Thyroxine enhances metabolic processes and the oxygen consumption. If the demands further increase, hypoxia can develop rapidly.

Five Causes of Hypoxemia (PaO$_2$)

The mechanisms that cause hypoxemia can be divided into those that increase PO$_2$ and those where PO$_2$ is preserved.

1. **Hypoventilation (low alveolar ventilation)**
   - PO$_2$ is normal
   - PaCO$_2$ is elevated (hypercapnia)
   - Increasing the fraction of inspired oxygen (FIO$_2$) can alleviate the hypoxemia and the hypercapnia can be corrected by mechanically ventilating the patient to eliminate CO$_2$.

- *Causes of Hypoventilation*
  - Depression of CNS by drugs, such as opiates or benzodiazepines
  - Inflammation, trauma, or hemorrhage in the brain stem
  - Abnormal spinal cord pathway
  - Disease of the motor neurons of the brain stem/spinal cord
  - Illness of the nerves supplying the respiratory muscles
  - Ailment of the neuromuscular junction
  - Disease of the respiratory muscles
  - Abnormality of the chest wall
  - Upper airway obstruction

2. **Low inspired oxygen (PIO$_2$)**

EXAMPLES OF LOW INSPIRED OXYGEN

- A decrease in barometric pressure (ie, breathing at high altitude)
- A decrease in FIO$_2$–accidental
- PaCO$_2$ is decreased. This reduction in PaCO$_2$ (hypocapnia) is due to hyperventilation in response to hypoxemia. Peripheral chemoreceptors sense the low arterial PO$_2$ and initiate an increase in ventilation through their input to the medullary respiratory center.

3. Right-to-left shunt

- PO_2 is elevated
- $PaCO_2$ is normal

Anatomic shunt: This occurs when a portion of blood bypasses the lungs through an anatomic channel.

- ***In healthy individuals***
    - a portion of the bronchial circulation's (blood supply to the conducting zone of the airways) venous blood drains into the pulmonary vein.
    - a portion of the coronary circulation's venous blood drains through the thebesian veins into the left ventricle.
- ***Congenital abnormalities***
    - intracardiac shunt (ie, tetralogy of Fallot: ventricular septal defect + pulmonary artery stenosis)
    - intrapulmonary fistulas (direct communication between a branch of the pulmonary artery and a pulmonary vein)

Physiologic shunt: In disease states, a portion of the cardiac output goes through the regular pulmonary vasculature but does not come into contact with alveolar air due to filling of the alveolar spaces with fluid (ie, pneumonia, drowning, pulmonary edema).

The key clinical feature of a right-left shunt is that the accompanying hypoxemia (low partial pressure of arterial oxygen) cannot be corrected with administration of supplemental O_2. This is because the shunted blood is not exposed to supplemental O_2 and remains low in O_2, lowering the overall arterial PO_2. This depression is marked because of the shape of the O_2 dissociation curve.

What Went Wrong?

If the amount of shunt is relatively small, useful gains in O_2 content of blood can be made by administering supplemental oxygen. For this reason, supplemental oxygen is never withheld from patients with hypoxemia.

4. Ventilation-perfusion dissimilarity is also known as ventilation-perfusion mismatch; both the symbols V/Q and VA/Q are often used in medical texts.

- $PaCO_2$ is normal
- PO_2 is elevated
- VA/Q inequality is the most common cause of hypoxemia in disease states

Alveolar ventilation brings O_2 into the lungs and removes CO_2 from it. Mixed venous blood brings CO_2 into the lungs and takes up alveolar oxygen.

The alveolar PO_2 and PCO_2 are determined by the relationship between alveolar ventilation and perfusion. Changing the ratio of alveolar ventilation to perfusion (VA/Q), will therefore change in the alveolar PO_2 and PCO_2. Alveolar ventilation is normally 4 to 6 L/min and pulmonary blood flow has a similar range. Therefore, the normal range of ventilation-perfusion ratio (VA/Q) for the whole lung is 0.8 to 1.2 L. Consider a hypothetical scenario where all the pulmonary blood flow is directed to the right lung and all the alveolar ventilation is directed to the left lung. Although the whole lung VA/Q ratio would be within the normal range, at the alveolar-capillary level there would be no gas exchange. Therefore, ventilation-perfusion must be matched at the individual alveolar-capillary level for gas exchange to be adequate. There are regional variations in the VA/Q ratio in the healthy upright lung. The VA/Q ratio decreases from the top to the bottom of the upright lung. This normal pattern accounts for approximately two-thirds of the normal PO_2 seen in healthy individuals and does not present any gas exchange problem. In disease states, there is a progression of disorganization in the normal pattern of VA/Q inequality.

5. **Diffusion impairment**

- $PaCO_2$ is normal
- PO_2 is normal at rest but may be elevated during exercise
  - a rare observation in the clinical setting
- In healthy individuals, the transit time for red blood cells in the pulmonary capillary exceeds that required for the PO_2 in the mixed venous blood to reach equilibrium with the alveolar gas. During exercise, when there is an increase blood flow, this transit time is decreased but there remains sufficient time for the PO_2 in the mixed venous blood to reach equilibrium with the alveolar gas. The exception to this is the elite athlete who achieves very high cardiac outputs during exercise resulting in a large decrement in pulmonary transit time.
- In disease states, impaired diffusion may occur when there is an increase in the thickness of the physical separation between alveolar gas and pulmonary capillary blood and a shortened pulmonary transit time. Both these conditions exist in a patient with an interstitial lung disease performing exercise.

What Went Wrong?

As a paramedic it is important to understand that hypoxemia refers to low partial pressures of O_2 in the blood and not low oxygen content of blood.

Factors related to hemoglobin, such as, anemia, hemoglobinopathies, and carbon monoxide poisoning are all factors that lower O_2 content. Stagnation of blood and histotoxic poisons such as cyanide, which lead to tissue hypoxia are not considered causes of hypoxemia since PaO_2 in these cases are normal. Understanding that there may be mixed causes of hypoxemia is often impossible to define in the acutely ill patient. In terms of treatment however the patient is always given supplemental oxygen with due caution.

REVIEW QUESTIONS

1. **There are four types of hypoxia, each of these having a number of possible causes. They include**

    A. hypoxic hypoxia

    B. anemic (hypemic) hypoxia

    C. stagnant hypoxia

    D. histotoxic hypoxia

    E. All the above

Correct answer is e.

2. **In right to left shunt the PO_2 is elevated and $PaCO_2$ is normal.**

    A. True

    B. False

Correct answer is a.

3. **While the blood's ability to pick up and transport O_2 may remain unaffected, a problem may also exist at the cellular level. An action by a toxic substance may prevent the diffusion of O_2 into the cells or may prevent the cells from utilizing oxygen. Cyanide is a poison which will cause this type of hypoxia.**

    A. Hypoxic hypoxia

    B. Anemic (hypemic) hypoxia

    C. Stagnant hypoxia

    D. Histotoxic hypoxia

Correct answer is d.

4. Any shock state in which there is widespread inadequate tissue perfusion, and hence inadequate tissue oxygenation. This form of hypoxia refers to end-organ perfusion. With this type of hypoxia, both the O_2 carrying capacity and the PO_2 may be normal. What causes this problem is an extreme blood flow deficit. This serious lack of blood flow may be localized to a specific region or may be generalized throughout the body.

   A. Hypoxic hypoxia
   B. Anemic (hypemic) hypoxia
   C. Stagnant hypoxia
   D. Histotoxic hypoxia

Correct answer is c.

5. In reduced or altered Hb, blood does not have a normal O_2 carrying capacity. There is either a reduced concentration of hemoglobin (anemia) or the Hb that is there, has a reduced ability to chemically unite with oxygen.

   A. Hypoxic hypoxia
   B. Anemic (hypemic) hypoxia
   C. Stagnant hypoxia
   D. Histotoxic hypoxia

Correct answer is b.

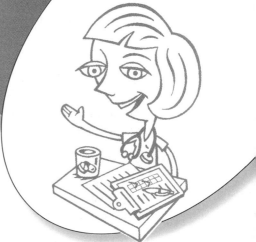

chapter 4

Pulse Oximetry and Capnography; What's the difference?

LEARNING OBJECTIVES

At the end of this chapter, you will be able to:

1. Define and describe end-tidal CO_2 ($ETCO_2$).
2. Describe methods of measuring $ETCO_2$.
3. Describe various clinical applications of $ETCO_2$.
4. Describe relationship between exhaled and arterial $ETCO_2$.
5. Identify common waveforms.
6. Define and describe pulse oximetry.
7. Describe methods of measuring pulse oximetry.

KEY TERMS

Alveolar-arterial gradient
Capnography
Carbon dioxide
Characteristics of a waveform
Dyshemoglobinemias
End-tidal CO_2

Mainstream
Oxygenation versus ventilation
$PaCO_2$ versus $PeTCO_2$
Pulse oximetry
Sidestream
Ventilation-perfusion relationship

Introduction

End-tidal CO_2 ($EtCO_2$) is the measurement of carbon dioxide (CO_2) in the airway at the end of each breath. Capnography provides a numeric reading (amount) and graphic display (waveform) of the $EtCO_2$ throughout the respiratory cycle. CO_2, produced by cells, is transported via the vascular system and diffused into the alveoli to be exhaled. $PaCO_2$, the partial pressure of CO_2 in arterial blood, is normally 2 to 5 mm Hg higher than $EtCO_2$ in the airway.

Capnography is the continuous, noninvasive measurement and graphical display of end-tidal carbon dioxide ($ETCO_2$). Capnography is an underutilized assessment tool in the management of respiratory patients. Determining endotracheal tube placement has become a significant issue in many health care environments. The technology of capnography provides an assessment tool for ventilation management.

Capnography was used originally in mechanically ventilated patients to assess patient levels of CO_2 on a breath-by-breath basis, continuously and noninvasively. The capnography sample chamber or sensor, placed between the patient's artificial airway and the ventilator, inspects the inhaled and exhaled gases for specific concentrations of CO_2. The inhaled and exhaled concentrations of CO_2 are graphically displayed as a waveform on the monitor, with a corresponding numerical value. Today, capnography plays a vital role in confirming intubation and verifying placement of an airway throughout intubation, ventilation assessment, and resuscitation. Hyperventilation often occurs preceding or following intubation. A real risk in continued hyperventilation is the associated cerebral vasoconstriction caused by the low level of CO_2.

What Went Wrong?

Although 100% oxygen (O_2) may have been used during initial resuscitation, providers should titrate inspired oxygen to the lowest level required to achieve an arterial oxygen saturation of ≥94%, so as to avoid potential oxygen toxicity. It is recognized that titration of inspired oxygen may not be possible immediately after out-of-hospital cardiac arrest until the patient is transported to the emergency department (ED) or, in the case of in-hospital arrest, the intensive care unit (ICU). Hyperventilation or "over-bagging" the patient is common after cardiac arrest and should be avoided because of potential adverse hemodynamic effects. Hyperventilation increases intrathoracic pressure and inversely lowers cardiac output. The decrease in $PaCO_2$ seen with hyperventilation can also potentially decrease cerebral blood flow directly. Ventilation may be started at 10 to 12 breaths per minute and titrated to achieve a $PETCO_2$ of 35 to 40 mm Hg or a $PaCO_2$ of 40 to 45 mm Hg.*

Various forms of capnography are available; enabling paramedics to identify problems with ventilation immediately. Capnography is also useful in monitoring nonintubated patients to assess ventilation and perfusion of the pulmonary vessels. The paramedic can use capnography as a supplemental tool and an early warning system to identify trends in ventilation and perfusion.

Carbon Dioxide (CO_2)

Carbon dioxide is the waste product of cellular metabolism. As cells consume oxygen, CO_2 is produced, which is transferred to the circulation, and delivered to the lungs via venous return. Cellular production of CO_2 is a metabolic by-product of the oxidative breakdown of metabolic fuels. The greater the metabolic rate, the higher the CO_2 production rate. Carbon dioxide dissolves rapidly in the cells and easily diffuses out of the cells and into the venous blood. Carbon dioxide is carried by the poorly oxygenated venous blood through the right heart and into the pulmonary arteries to reach the capillaries surrounding each pulmonary alveolus.

As ambient air is drawn into the alveolus during inspiration, the CO_2 in the blood diffuses through the capillary and alveolar walls into the alveolar air sac.

---

*Peberdy MA, Callaway CW, Neumar RW, Geocadin RG, Zimmerman JL, Donnino M, Gabrielli A, Silvers SM, Zaritsky AL, Merchant R, Vanden Hoek TL, Kronick SL. Part 9: post–cardiac arrest care: 2010 American Heart Association Guidelines for Cardiopulmonary Resuscitation and Emergency Cardiovascular Care. Circulation. 2010; 122(suppl 3): S768–S786.

Under normal conditions, one pass of the blood through the alveolar capillary drives the alveolar PCO_2 nearly to match (usually within 5 mm Hg) the $PaCO_2$. As expiration begins, the gas containing carbon dioxide is expelled from the alveoli to displace and mix with the air in the bronchial tree. As this mixture of gases reaches the upper airways and the capnography monitor, the measured PCO_2 rises sharply to a plateau and then slowly increases to a peak as the CO_2 level continues to increase. This peak PCO_2 at the end of expiration is known as the $ETCO_2$; in healthy individuals, it is generally within 5 mm Hg of the $PaCO_2$. These differences can be affected by many patient factors, increasing, for example, in patients undergoing aggressive emergency procedures and in patients with significant cardiopulmonary disease.

Once inspiration begins, the PCO_2 measured at the mouth or nose drops rapidly to almost zero. The rapid expiratory rise, slowly rising plateau, and drastic decrease at the beginning of inspiration constitute the characteristic waveform of the capnogram. The importance of the $ETCO_2$ waveform and numerical value resides in their ability to reflect the cardiopulmonary status of the patient. A capnograph ($ETCO_2$ monitor) provides this information to the pre-hospital clinician continuously.

Excretion of CO_2 is the final common pathway of metabolism, and it provides a useful global indication of patient status. Ventilation must be adequate to carry oxygen into the lungs.

Oxygen is supplied into the erythrocytes and transported to the cells at the tissue level. Transport is a function of the cardiovascular system. The process of aerobic metabolism consumes the oxygen and produces CO_2. The carbon dioxide is transferred from the tissue into the red blood cells and is transported to the lungs for elimination. Hypoxemia, cerebral ischemia, and coronary ischemia are possible even in the presence of normal capnography waveforms and numerical values.

The capnograph uses infrared light technology that incorporates a very sensitive emitter and a detector that identifies only the light-absorption signal of CO_2. This specificity for carbon dioxide allows the use of capnography in the presence of other gases or aerosolized medications. The accuracy of $ETCO_2$ measurements can be confirmed using the waveform identifying the unique shape of the characteristic capnogram. Newer devices allow for accurate monitoring even with high respiration rates and respiratory low tidal volumes, as are often present in neonatal and pediatric patients.

Oxygenation versus Ventilation

Oxygenation is how we get oxygen to the tissue. Oxygen is inhaled into the lungs where gas exchange occurs at the capillary-alveolar membrane.

Oxygen is transported to the tissues through the bloodstream. Pulse oximetry measures oxygenation. At the cellular level, oxygen and glucose combine to produce energy. Carbon dioxide, a waste product of this process (The Krebs cycle), diffuses into the blood. Ventilation (the movement of air) is how we get rid of CO_2. Carbon dioxide is carried back through the blood and exhaled by the lungs through the alveoli. Capnography measures ventilation (Figure 4-1).

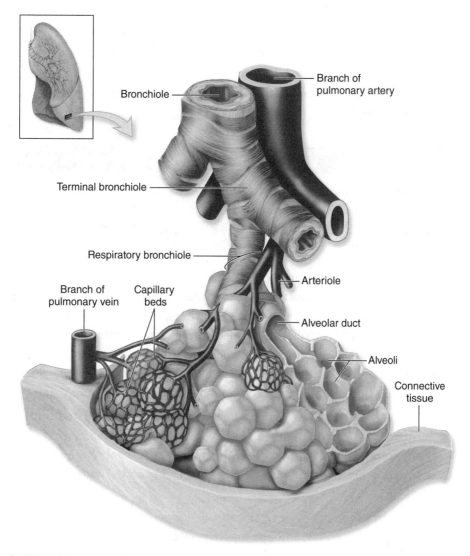

FIGURE 4-1 · Alveolar capillary junction.

Reproduced with permission from McKinley M, Dean O'Loughlin V. *Human Anatomy*. 2nd ed. ISBN 978-0-07-296549-0. Page 758.

Alveolar-Arterial Gradient

Observing the difference between arterial and exhaled CO_2 can also give valuable data about the patient's condition. The alveolar-arterial gradient is the difference between the alveolar carbon dioxide level ($ETCO_2$) and the arterial level.

- Normal $PaCO_2$ is 35 to 45 mm Hg.
- In adults with normal cardiorespiratory function (normal ventilation and perfusion) the $ETCO_2$ is 2 to 5 mm Hg lower than the $PaCO_2$, this is generally due to alveolar mixing.
- In infants and small children the gradient is lower and closely reflects $PaCO_2$ (<3 mm Hg). This is because of better V/Q matching and hence a lower alveolar dead space.

The gradient can vary from patient to patient and at times the $ETCO_2$ may be higher than the $PaCO_2$.

EXAMPLES

- Healthy subjects with large tidal volumes and low frequency ventilation
- In pregnant women

Ventilation-Perfusion Relationship

Ventilation in the alveoli must be properly matched with blood perfusion in the pulmonary capillaries for adequate gas exchange to occur. The ventilation-perfusion ratio (V/Q) describes the relationship between airflow in the alveoli and blood flow in the pulmonary capillaries. If ventilation is perfectly matched to perfusion, the V/Q is 1. Both ventilation and perfusion are unevenly distributed throughout the normal lung. The normal V/Q is 0.8.

- Dead space ventilation occurs when the alveoli are ventilated but not perfused. Clinical situations such as hypotension, hypovolemia, excessive positive end-expiratory pressure (PEEP), pulmonary embolism, or cardiopulmonary arrest result in a decreased $ETCO_2$ and a widening of the gradient.
- Shunt perfusion occurs when the alveoli are perfused but not ventilated. This can be due to pneumonia, mucous plugging, and atelectasis. $ETCO_2$ may decrease slightly, but carbon dioxide is highly soluble and will diffuse out of the blood into the available alveoli. Therefore, little effect on the gradient is seen. In this case, the patient's oxygenation status may suffer,

and PEEP or continuous positive airway pressure will be indicated to re-expand the atelectatic lung units.

Capnography versus Pulse Oximetry

Capnography provides an immediate picture of patient's condition. Pulse oximetry is delayed.

Hold your breath. Capnography will show immediate apnea, while pulse oximetry will show a high saturation for several minutes.

Circulation and Metabolism

While capnography is a direct measurement of ventilation in the lungs; it also indirectly measures metabolism and circulation. For example, an increased metabolism will increase the production of carbon dioxide increasing the $ETCO_2$. A decrease in cardiac output will lower the supply of CO_2 to the lungs decreasing the $ETCO_2$.

$PaCO_2$ versus $PeTCO_2$

$PaCO_2$ equals partial pressure of carbon dioxide in arterial blood gases (ABG). The $PaCO_2$ is measured by drawing the ABGs, which also measure the arterial pH. If ventilation and perfusion are stable, $PaCO_2$ should correlate to $PetCO_2$.

Connecting the Endotracheal Tube to Capnography

Respiratory gases are analyzed by two possible methods:

- Sidestream
- Mainstream

Sidestream analysis: Sample of respiratory gas is withdrawn continuously throughout respiratory cycle and sampled in an analyzer contained within main unit. Units typically have a 1.0-2.0-mm small-bore pipe leading from endotracheal (ET) tube to the main unit.

Mainstream analysis: Gas is analyzed as it passes through sensor at the end of ET tube. Sensor is connected to the main unit by a cable. CO_2 concentration is assessed as patient breathes through sensor.

Clinical Uses of Capnography

How can such an understanding of a capnogram aid in more effective pre-hospital care? There are several clinical applications.

- Intubation verification: This is the most common problem with airway management and ventilation can be detected using capnography.

The American Heart Association has identified capnography as a tool for secondary confirmation of intubation. Pediatric advanced life support (PALS) also calls for the use of $ETCO_2$ to confirm ET placement for all patients with a perfusing rhythm.

- Transportation: It is recommended that capnography be used during transportation of ventilated patients to immediately identify ET dislodgement. $ETCO_2$ should also be used continuously to monitor the intubated pediatric patients due to a higher, more anterior glottic opening and a shorter trachea which makes dislodgement of the tube more likely. Capnography can also assist in determining proper ventilation with bag-valve-mask devices when hyper or hypoventilation is common. Transferring a mechanically ventilated or pulmonary-challenged patient to other diagnostic departments within the hospital involves extra attention. These high risk patients should be given a real-time, breath-to-breath pulmonary assessment that only capnography can provide.

- CPR: Capnography is a valuable tool during cardiopulmonary resuscitation (CPR). CO_2 levels fall abruptly because of the absence of cardiac output (blood flow) and pulmonary blood flow. Studies have shown the closer to normal the $ETCO_2$ levels are the more effective cardiac output is during resuscitation. Lower $ETCO_2$ levels observed during resuscitation may signal a need for changes in CPR techniques (rate/depth/force) of compression.

- Predictor of death/survival: Capnography can confirm the futility of resuscitation. A study in the *New England Journal of Medicine* concluded that an $ETCO_2$ level of 10 mm Hg or less measured 20 minutes after the initiation of advanced cardiac life support accurately predicts death in patients with cardiac arrest associated with electrical activity but no pulse.

Cardiopulmonary resuscitation may be terminated in such patients. Likewise, case studies have shown that patients with high initial $EtCO_2$ reading were more likely to be resuscitated than those who didn't. The greater the initial value, the likelier the chance of a successful resuscitation. Principles of capnography used with cardiac arrest patients include the following:

- Patients in cardiac arrest will generally have low $EtCO_2$ values because perfusion is poor. CPR offers roughly 30% of normal circulation, producing only one-third the normal exhaled CO_2. In patients receiving good cardiac compressions, the value will be slightly higher. As rescuers tire, end-tidal values decrease—a good indication of when it is time to switch compressors. As a fresh rescuer takes over, you should see $EtCO_2$ levels rise.

- Patients with return of spontaneous circulation (ROSC) often have a rapid rise in $EtCO_2$ values several minutes before pulses become palpable. Metabolism is to CO_2 what your thermostat is to your house. The higher you turn it up, the more production you get. As the patient's own metabolism kicks in and excess CO_2 is washed out of previously under perfused tissue, the value will rise.

- In cardiac arrest patients with sustained $ETCO_2$ values of 10 mm Hg or less despite advanced cardiac life support (ACLS) therapy, resuscitation can be stopped. These patients are clinically dead, and a study found an $EtCO_2$ cutoff of 10 made the difference between survivors and non-survivors both dramatic and obvious.

- $ETCO_2$ can be used to assess the severity of an asthma/COPD exacerbation and the effectiveness of intervention. Bronchospasm will produce a characteristic "shark fin" wave form, as the patient has to struggle to exhale. Asthma values change with severity. With mild asthma the CO_2 will drop (<35 mm Hg) as the patient hyperventilates to compensate. As the asthma becomes severe, and the patient is tiring and has little air movement, the CO_2 numbers will rise to dangerous levels (>60 mm Hg). If treatment is successful the "shark fin" will be eliminated and return the $ETCO_2$ levels to normal or near normal.

- Hyperventilation can increase blood pressure, and, with head injury patients, increased blood pressure can exacerbate cerebral edema. Monitoring of $ETCO_2$ can assist the paramedic in maintaining stable CO_2 levels, thus avoiding secondary injury from accidental increased cerebral edema.

- In most patients the $ETCO_2$ correlates well with the $PaCO_2$. Understanding this, capnography can function as an excellent adjunct to other monitoring methods, including ABG analysis and oximetry. While $ETCO_2$ levels in very ill patients should be interpreted with caution, trends in $ETCO_2$ correlate with changes in the $PaCO_2$ and can provide an early warning of metabolic or cardiorespiratory problems such as shunting, dead space, bronchoconstriction, or pulmonary embolism. Capnography allows for the trending of the $ETCO_2$ value and its subsequent comparison with ABG values.

- Capnography can assist the in-hospital clinician in successful ventilator weaning ensuring that the patient is clinically stable and without clinically significant residual effect of any anesthetic agents or sedatives. When $ETCO_2$ values are considered in combination with standard weaning criteria/parameters, the chance of a successful extubation increases. $ETCO_2$ value during weaning can indicate if the patient is experiencing a hypercapnic episode and may decrease the number of ABGs needed. "Some clinicians utilized $ETCO_2$ as a marker of the metabolic rate and, therefore, as a way of determining optimal ventilator settings during the weaning process." Patients with higher metabolic rates (ie, sepsis) may be difficult to wean under these conditions making it often difficult to predict the success of weaning.

- $ETCO_2$ can provide an early warning sign of shock. A patient with a sudden drop in cardiac output will show a drop in the $ETCO_2$ numbers that may be regardless of any change in breathing. "A patient with low cardiac output caused by cardiogenic shock or hypovolemia resulting from hemorrhage won't carry as much CO_2 per minute back to the lungs to be exhales. This patient's $ETCO_2$ will be reduced. It doesn't necessarily mean the patient is hyperventilating or that their arterial CO_2 level will be reduced. Reduced perfusion to the lungs alone causes this phenomenon. The patient's lung function may be perfectly normal.

Different Sampling Mechanisms Have Differing Implications for Their Use

To use capnography we must understand the wave form and the information given by the waveform. The positive deflection of the wave represents the exhalation of the patient. The top of the wave represent the alveolar plateau and the end of the elevated wave represent the $ETCO_2$. The sharp drop of the wave represents the inhalation stage. The normal range is between 35 and 45 mm Hg (Figure 4-2).

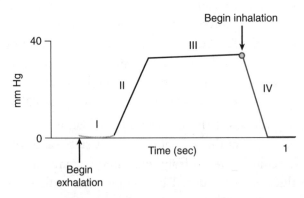

FIGURE 4-2 · Reproduced with permission from Brauss B, Hess DR: *Capnography for procedural sedation and analgesia in the emergency department. Ann Emerg Med 50: 172, 2007 (Table 1, p. 176).*

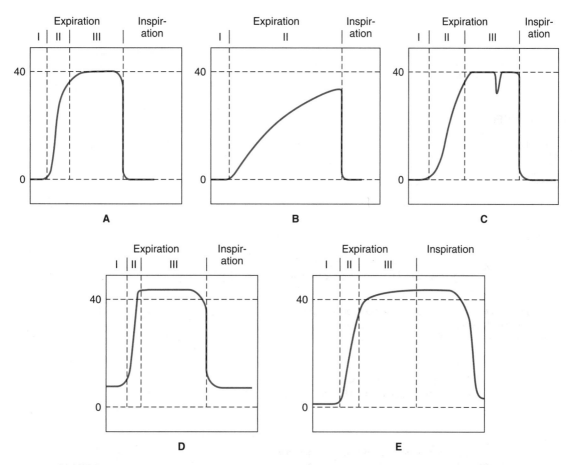

FIGURE 4-3 · Reproduced with permission from Morgan, Jr. GE, Mikhail MS, Murray MJ, eds. *Clinical Anesthesiology.* 4th ed. 2006. New York: Copyright © McGraw-Hill Education. All rights reserved.

There is a large amount of information that can be gathered by the waveform. The amplitude of the wave will tell you how much oxygen exchange is occurring and the wave configuration tells you the quality of the respiration. Let's consider some of the waveforms and see what information is being provided to us (Figure 4-3).

Five characteristics of a waveform are as follows (Figure 4-4):

1. Frequency
2. Rhythm
3. Height:
    a. hyperventilation—decreased height (low CO_2)
    b. hypoventilation—increased height (high CO_2)
4. Baseline
5. Shape—identical to all humans with healthy lungs

Waveform Analysis:

NORMAL
"Square box" waveform; baseline CO_2 = 0; $ETCO_2$ = 35–45 mmHg
Management: Monitor

DISLODGED ETT
Loss of waveform, Loss of $ETCO_2$ reading
Management: Replace ETT

ESOPHAGEAL INTUBATION
Absence of waveform, Absence of detectable $ETCO_2$
Management: Re-intubate

CPR
"Square box" waveform; baseline CO_2 = 0; $ETCO_2$ = 10–15 mmHg
(possibly higher) with adequate CPR
Management: Change rescuers if $ETCO_2$ drops < 10 mmHg

BRONCHOSPASM
"Sharkfin" pattern with/without prolonged expiration (asthma,
COPD, allergic reaction:
Management: Bronchodilators

ROSC
As in CPR, but $ETCO_2$ rises above 10–15 mmHg
Management: Check for pulse; contact BIOTEL for drip
authorization

RISING BASELINE
Patient is rebreathing CO_2
Management: Check equipment for adequate oxygen inflow
Allow intubated patient more time to exhale

HYPOVENTILATION
Prolonged waveform; baseline CO_2 = 0; $ETCO_2$ > 45 mmHg
Management: Assist ventilations or intubate, if needed

HYPERVENTILATION
Shortened waveform; baseline $ETCO_2$ = 0; $ETCO_2$ < 35 mmHg
Management: Biofeedback if conscious; assisted ventilation rate
if unconscious/intubated

PATIENT BREATHING AROUND ET TUBE
Angled, sloping downstroke on waveform
Adult: Broken cuff or tube is too small
Pediatric: tube is too small
Management: Assess patient, oxygenation, ventilation;
may need to reintubate

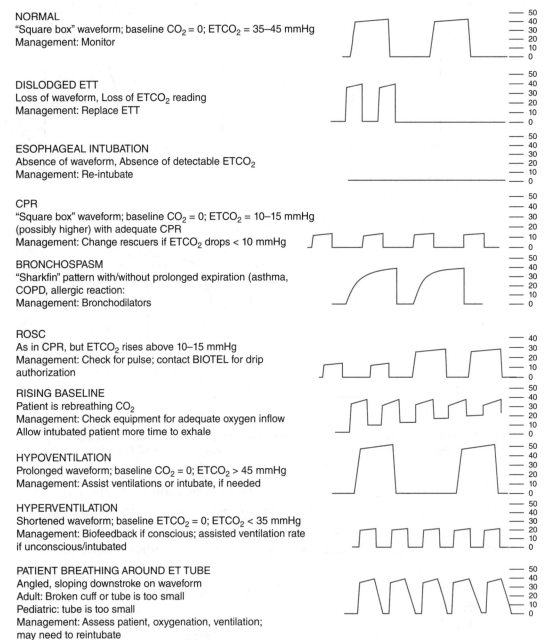

FIGURE 4-4 • Waveform analysis.
Courtesy of UT Southwestern Medical Center at Dallas / BioTel EMS System, Protocols for Therapy.
Reproduced with permisssion from UT Southwestern Medical Center at Dallas / BioTel EMS System,
Protocols for Therapy, July 1, 2003.

Principles of Pulse Oximetry

Introduction

Blood oxygen content is now considered the "fifth vital sign"; joining temperature, respiratory rate, heart rate, and blood pressure. One of the main advantages of pulse oximetry is that measurements are taken noninvasively through optical measurements.

A pulse oximeter measures and displays the pulse rate and the saturation of hemoglobin (Hb) in arterial blood. This saturation of Hb is a measure of the average amount of O_2 bound to each hemoglobin molecule. The absorption of visible light by a hemoglobin solution varies with oxygenation.

Pulse oximetry is based on two physical principles: (a) the presence of a pulsatile signal generated by arterial blood, which is relatively independent of nonpulsatile arterial blood, venous and capillary blood, and other tissues; and (b) the fact that oxyhemoglobin (O_2 Hb) and reduced Hb have different absorption spectra.

The chemical binding of different types of Hb species changes the physical properties of the hemoglobin as well. The oxygen which is chemically combined with hemoglobin inside the RBCs makes up nearly all of the oxygen present in blood (there is also a very small amount which is dissolved in the plasma). Oxygen saturation, which is often referred to as SaO_2 or SpO_2, is defined as the ratio of oxyhemoglobin (HbO_2) to the total concentration of hemoglobin present in the blood.

Accuracy versus Saturation

Accuracy at different levels of oxygen saturation is not the same. Oxygen saturation is divided into three ranges:

- Normal saturation
- High saturation
- Hypoxic condition (low saturation level)

Normal Saturation (90% to 97.5%)

Most models of pulse oximeters have a reliable performance in this range, and are well calibrated in this range since it is the most commonly found condition.

High Saturation (> 97.5%)

Pulse oximeters are designed to give a saturation reading of less than or equal to 100%; this limits the potential for positive errors and makes precision calculations difficult to interpret in this high range. As long as the oxygen saturation is over 97%, the patients are in favorable conditions and they require no urgent medical attention.

Low Saturation (< 80%)

Ethically manufacturers cannot stimulate severe hypoxia repeatedly in volunteers for calibration purposes. For this reason mainly, pulse oximeters have a high potential for errors at low saturations. The error associated with low saturations can be explained by a reduction on the signal-to-noise ratio in pulse oximetry. As level of saturation decreases, less red light is able to penetrate through the tissues due to a high absorbance of Hb, so the alternating current (AC) signal becomes weaker. To compensate for this drawback, the LED-driving current and the photodiode amplifier gain are increased to maintain the AC signal in a usual range. As the gain increases, incidental electrical and physiological noise also increase, therefore resulting in a decline in the pulse oximeters accuracy.

Dyshemoglobinemias

The accuracy of pulse oximetry is excellent when the oxygen saturation is between the ranges of 70% and 100%, provided the only hemoglobin species present in the blood are reduced hemoglobin and oxygenated hemoglobin. If carboxyhemoglobin (COHb) or methemoglobin (MetHb) is present in significant amounts, the accuracy should be questioned. COHb and MetHb also absorb light at the pulse oximeter's two wavelengths, and this leads to an error. MetHb occurs when the normal ferrous (Fe^{2+}) state of the iron in Hb is oxidized to the ferric state (Fe^{3+}). MetHb absorbs equal amounts of red and near infrared light. The ratio of pulsatile and nonpulsatile absorbance in the two wavelengths is equal to 1 at a hemoglobin oxygen saturation of 85%. A high concentration of MetHb causes the saturation to approximate 85%. When the patient is hypoxic (saturation 40%-50%), the MetHb artificially increases the pulse oximeter reading to 85%. Conversely, if the oxygen saturation is 100%, the MetHb spuriously decreases the pulse oximeter reading to 85%. This explains why the pulse oximeter reading stay sat 85% in the presence of significant methemoglobinemia, regardless of the "true" oxygen saturation, while a multiwavelength cooximeter will show decreasing oxygen saturations at increasing MetHb levels. Whenever significant methemoglobinemia is suspected, it is imperative to check an arterial blood sample in a cooximeter to measure the amount of oxyhemoglobin and methemoglobin. The treatment of methemoglobinemia with methylene blue further confuses the picture, as the dye lowers the pulse oximeter reading as well. Once the MetHb level is reduced, and the methylene blue is diluted or excreted in the urine, the saturation measured by pulse oximetry returns to normal. Carboxyhemoglobin levels in nonsmokers are less than 2%, while they may be as high as 10% to 20% in heavy smokers. COHb absorbs very little light at 940 nm, while at 660 nm its extinction coefficient is very similar to oxyhemoglobin. Thus the presence of significant COHb will resemble the curve of oxyhemoglobin in the red range, with no effect on the infrared, and "look like" oxyhemoglobin, causing the pulse oximeter to over read. For every 1% of circulating carboxyhemoglobin, the pulse oximeter over reads by 1%. Fifty percent of cigarette smokers have a carboxyhemoglobin concentration of 6%. When the presence of either of these dyshemoglobins is suspected, pulse oximetry should be supplemented. Other common sources of error include extraneous energy sources, especially bright visible or infrared light which may flood or overload the semiconductor detector, and display a value of 85%. The problem of bright fluorescent ambient light causing false readings can be reduced by covering the sensor with felt pads. Pulsatile veins cause under reading as the oximeter cannot differentiate between pulsatile arteries and veins. Tricuspid regurgitation and neonates with hyperdynamic circulation may have inaccurate readings.

Poor Function with Poor Perfusion

In addition to artifacts and misreading, there is asmall but definite incidence of failure with pulse oximetry. The most important limitation of pulse oximeters is that they are inaccurate in patients who need them the most. As it is mandatory to have a good pulse waveform (this is essential for the oximeter to calculate the ratio of pulsatile to nonpulsatile absorbance and derive the oxygen saturation), the pulse oximeter fails to give accurate readings whenever the peripheral pulsations are poor. Adequate arterial pulsations are required to distinguish the light absorbed by arterial blood from that absorbed by venous blood and tissue and readings may be unreliable or unavailable if there is loss or diminution of the peripheral pulse (proximal blood pressure cuff inflation, leaning on an extremity, improper positioning, hypotension, hypothermia, cardiopulmonary bypass, low cardiac output, hypovolemia, peripheral vascular disease or infusion of vasoactive drugs). A Valsalva maneuver as seen in laboring patients will cause a decrease in pulse amplitude, which adversely affects the oximeter's ability to provide useful data. Cold extremities may impair the functioning of the pulse oximeter especially if the patient has Raynaud's phenomenon. Under these conditions, some pulse oximeters blank the display or give a message such as low quality signal or inadequate signal. Others freeze the display at the previous reading when they are unable to detect a consistent pulse wave.

What Went Wrong?

Raynaud's disease is more than simply having cold hands and cold feet, and it's not the same as frostbite. Signs and symptoms of Raynaud's depend on the frequency, duration, and severity of the blood vessel spasms that underlie the disorder. Raynaud's disease symptoms include:

- Cold fingers and toes
- Sequence of color changes in the skin in response to cold or stress
- Numb, prickly feeling or stinging pain upon warming or relief of stress

During an attack of Raynaud's, affected areas of the skin usually turn white at first. Then, the affected areas often turn blue, feel cold and numb, and sense of touch is dulled. As circulation improves, the affected areas may turn red, throb, tingle, or swell. The order of the changes of color isn't the same for all people, and not everyone experiences all three colors. Occasionally, an attack affects just one or two fingers or toes. Attacks don't necessarily always affect the same digits. Although Raynaud's most commonly affects fingers and toes, the condition can also affect other areas of the body, such as nose, lips, ears, and even nipples. An attack may last less than a minute to several hours. People who suffer from Raynaud's accompanied by another disease will likely also have signs and symptoms related to their basic underlying condition.

The presence of a functioning pulse oximeter should not be construed as evidence of adequate tissue oxygenation or oxygen delivery to vital organs. Warming cool extremities may increase the pulse amplitude, provided the cardiac output is not depressed. The actual failure rate varies with the individual monitor and is increased with ear and nose sensors. Monitors that can analyze the signal and reject artifacts have fewer episodes of failure. Pulse oximeters with signal extraction technology may perform better during low perfusion states. Pulse oximeters are most unreliable in the newborn, as minor changes in skin temperature, as well as minor adjustments in contact can cause motion artifacts and a poor signal.

Difficulty in Detecting High Oxygen Partial Pressures

At high saturations, small changes in saturation are associated with relatively large changes in PaO_2. Thus the pulse oximeter has a limited ability to distinguish high but safe levels of arterial oxygen from excess oxygenation, which may be harmful, as in premature newborns or patients with severe COPD who use the hypoxic drive to breathe.

Delayed Detection of Hypoxic Events

While the response time of the pulse oximeter is generally fast, there may be a significant delay between a change in alveolar oxygen tension and a change in the oximeter reading. It is possible for arterial oxygen to reach dangerous levels before the pulse oximeter alarm is activated.

Delay in response is related to sensor location. Desaturation is detected earlier when the sensor is placed more centrally. Lag time will be increased with poor perfusion and a decrease in blood flow to the site monitored. Performance of a neural block may cause the lag time to decrease while venous obstruction, peripheral vasoconstriction, hypothermia, and motion artifacts delay detection of hypoxemia. Increasing the time over which the pulse signals are averaged also increases the delay time.

Erratic Performance with Irregular Rhythms

Irregular heart rhythms can cause erratic performance. During aortic balloon pulsation, the augmentation of diastolic pressure exceeds that of systolic pressure. This leads to a double or triple-packed arterial pressure waveform that confuses the pulse oximeter so that it may not provide a reading. Pulse oximetry is notoriously unreliable in the presence of rapid atrial fibrillation.

Nail Polish and Coverings

Some shades of black, blue, and green nail polish may cause significantly lower saturation readings. Synthetic nails may also interfere with pulse oximetry readings. One way to overcome this problem is to orient the probe so it transmits light from one side of the finger to the other side. The presence of onychomycosis, a yellowish gray color caused by fungus can cause falsely low SpO_2 readings. Dirt under the nail can also cause difficulty in obtaining reliable readings.

Although there is one report of dried blood on a finger causing erroneou slow saturation readings, other authors have found that dried blood does not affect the accuracy of the pulse oximeter.

Loss of Accuracy at Low Values

Measurement of SpO_2 is less accurate at low values, and 70% saturation is generally taken as the lowest accurate reading.

Motion Artifacts

Motion of the sensor relative to the skin can cause an artifact that the pulse oximeter is unable to differentiate from normal arterial pulsations. Motion may produce a prolongation in the detection time for hypoxemia without giving a warning. Motion is usually a problem during EMS care; but if the patient is shivering, moving about (as during inhalation induction of smallchildren), or being transported it can be significant. The ability of an oximeter to deal with motion artifacts depends on the correlation with the onset of the motion and the start of monitoring. If the motion precedes the onset of monitoring, there is a greater decrement in performance. Motion artifacts can usually be recognized by false or erratic pulse rate displays or distorted plethysmographic waveforms. Increased pulse amplitude is an indicator of movement but not necessarily of artificial SpO_2 readings. Artifacts caused by motion can be decreased by careful sensor positioning on a different extremity from that being stimulated. Ear, cheek and nose probes may be more useful than finger probes in restless patients, and flexible probes that are taped in place, or probes lined with soft material are less susceptible to motion artifacts than clip-on probes. Neonates and children with their tiny digits and poor contact with probes are most susceptible to motion artifact. Pulse oximeters vary in their ability to identify readings associated with movement. Lengthening the averaging mode will increase the likelihood that enough true pulses will be detected to reject motion artifacts. Some manufacturers use the R-wave of the patient's ECG to synchronize the optical measurement. Oximeters with signal extraction technology which use mathematical manipulation of the oximeter's light signals to measure and subtract the noise components associated with motion-will have fewer artifacts.

Pressure on the Sensor

Pressure on the sensor may result in inaccurate SpO_2 readings without affecting pulse rate determination.

Hyperemia

If a limb is hyperemic, the flow of capillary and venous blood becomes pulsatile. In this situation the absorption of light from these sources will be included in the saturation computations with resulting decrease inaccuracy of the oxygen saturation measured by pulse oximetry. A pulse oximeter placed near the site of blood transfusion may show transient decreases in oxygen saturation with rapid infusion of the blood.

Failure to Detect Absence of Circulation

A pulse oximeter signal and a normal reading do not necessarily imply adequacy of tissue perfusion. Some pulse oximeters show a pulse despite inadequate tissueperfusion or even when no pulse is present, as ambient light may produce a false signal.

Discrepancies in Readings from Different Monitors

A discrepancy in readings between difference brands of oximeters on the same patient at the same time is not uncommon. One reason for this is differences in methods of calibration and the variation in the time it takes various monitors to detect desaturation.

Failure to Detect Hypoventilation

Hypoventilation and hypercarbia may occur without a decrease in hemoglobin oxygen saturation, especially if the patient is receiving supplemental oxygen. Pulse oximetry should not be relied upon to assess the adequacy of ventilation or to detect disconnections or esophageal intubations. A capnograph is necessary to detect these complications. It is important to realize that while a capnograph detects esophageal intubation or a disconnection, pulse oximetry detects only the effects of such a mishap, namely, hypoxia, and valuable time maybe lost before taking corrective measures. In summary, pulse oximeters are poorly calibrated for saturations below 80%, and in general, accuracy and precision are worse for saturations above this percentage.

REVIEW QUESTIONS

1. **The advantages of mainstream capnography include a faster response time and intrinsically is more accurate.**
   A. True
   B. False

Correct answer is a.

2. The normal value of $ETCO_2$ is:

   A. below 30 mm Hg.
   B. above 50 mm Hg.
   C. between 35 and 45 mm Hg.
   D. 120/80 mm Hg.

Correct answer is c.

3. The process of getting O_2 to the tissues is known as:

   A. oxygenation.
   B. ventilation.
   C. Both a and b.
   D. None of the above.

Correct answer is a.

4. Sudden loss of $EtCO_2$ to zero or near zero indicates immediate danger because no respiration is detected. Possible causes include:

   A. esophageal intubation.
   B. complete airway disconnect from ventilator.
   C. complete ventilator malfunction.
   D. obstructed endotracheal tube.
   E. All of the above are correct.

Correct answer is e.

5. The respiratory process consists of all of the following except:

   A. cellular metabolism of food into energy—O_2 consumption and CO_2 production.
   B. transport of O_2 and CO_2 between cells and pulmonary capillaries, and diffusion from/into alveoli.
   C. ventilation between alveoli and atmosphere.
   D. All of the above are correct.

Correct answer is d.

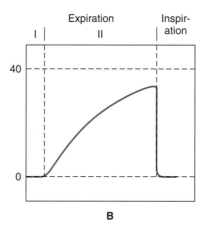

FIGURE 4-5 •

6. The above figure depicts a patient with:

A. curare cleft.

B. severe chronic obstructive pulmonary disease.

C. a normal capnogram.

D. None of the above.

Correct answer is b.

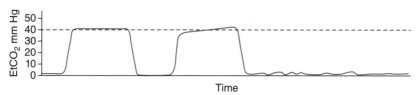

FIGURE 4-6 • Reproduced with permission from County of Buncombe, Emergency Medical Service, 60 Court Plaza, Asheville, N.C. 28801-3561.
Accessed website: http://emsstaff.buncombecounty.org/inhousetraining/capnography/part-2/default.asp; January 21, 2013. Self-study online BCEMS website.

7. You are treating a trauma patient who has an advanced airway in place. The capnogram in Figure 4-6 is an indicator that there is a problem with the airway. What is the possible causes:

A. Patient has spontaneous breathing.

B. Bronchospasm.

C. The airway may have become displaced or obstructed.

D. Head trauma with herniation.

Correct answer is c.

8. **Each part of the capnography waveform represents a different phase of the respiratory cycle. Phase I represents:**

   A. respiratory baseline, CO_2 free dead space air, normally 0.

   B. expiratory pp stroke, rapid rise due to mixing of dead space air and alveolar air, should be steep.

   C. expiratory plateau, exhalation of mostly alveolar air.

   D. inspiratory down-stroke, inhalation of CO_2 free gas, quickly returns to the baseline.

Correct answer is a.

9. **Each part of the capnography waveform represents a different phase of the respiratory cycle. Phase III represents:**

   A. respiratory baseline, CO_2 free dead space air, normally 0.

   B. expiratory upstroke, rapid rise due to mixing of dead space air and alveolar air, should be steep.

   C. expiratory plateau, exhalation of mostly alveolar air.

   D. inspiratory down-stroke, inhalation of CO_2 free gas, quickly returns to the baseline.

Correct answer is c.

10. **Each part of the capnography waveform represents a different phase of the respiratory cycle. Phase IV represents:**

   A. respiratory baseline, CO_2 free dead space air, normally 0.

   B. expiratory upstroke, rapid rise due to mixing of dead space air and alveolar air, should be steep.

   C. expiratory plateau, exhalation of mostly alveolar air.

   D. inspiratory down-stroke, inhalation of CO_2 free gas, quickly returns to the baseline.

Correct answer is d.

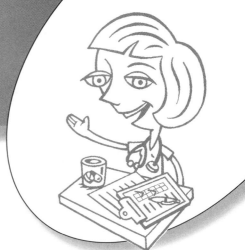

chapter 5

Oxygen Delivery Devices and Bag-Valve-Mask Ventilation

LEARNING OBJECTIVES

At the end of this chapter, you will be able to:

1. Describe the basic function of the respiratory system.

2. Explain the importance of oxygen use.

3. Identify indications (signs) of oxygen use.

4. Identify devices used to supply oxygen.

KEY TERMS

Aerosol mask
Bag-valve mask
Diffusion
Nasal prongs
Non-rebreather mask

Oxygen dissociation
Partial pressures
Tidal volumes
Vapor pressure

Introduction

Oxygen is an essential ingredient of life. The human body depends on oxygen to live. Chapter 1 examines both the anatomical and physiological aspects of the respiratory system important in pulmonary mechanics and ventilation. This chapter is intended to be a continuation of the discussion on the respiratory system focusing on the principles of gas transport, factors affecting transport, the chemical control of the respiration, and the practical application and usage of oxygen delivery systems.

The air we breathe consists of 21% oxygen. The oxygen level in the air is adequate for most people. However, when a person has low oxygen levels, supplemental oxygen is required. Oxygen therapy is the administration of oxygen to increase the supply of oxygen to the lungs.

The aim of oxygen therapy is to relieve hypoxia (deficiencies of oxygen at the tissue level), decrease the work of breathing, and decrease the workload of the heart.

Partial Pressures

Gas molecules are in fluid motion all around us. The earth's atmosphere is made up of many different gases, each one comprising a certain percentage of the total amount.

Like other molecules, gases have weight and create a downward force as a result of the earth's gravity. The total downward force of these gases is known as atmospheric pressure.

At sea level, this downward pressure is sufficient to support a column of mercury (Hg) 760 millimeters (mm) high. 1 atmosphere is equal to 760 mm Hg. Gases are also measured in "torr" units. One torr unit equals 1 mm Hg. Thus:

$$1 \text{ atmosphere} = 760 \text{ mm Hg} = 760 \text{ torr}$$

$$\boxed{\begin{array}{c} a\,b\,b\,b\,b \\ b\,a\,b\,b\,b \end{array}} = 760 \text{ mm Hg}$$

Figure 5-1 • P_T of two gases.

It is often important to calculate the pressure of a single gas in a mixture. This value is known as the partial pressure (often called the tension) of that gas. The partial pressure (P) of any gas is the pressure which it would exert if it were alone and unaffected by changes in other gases. There are a number of gas laws which help summarize the behavior of gases. Relevant to this discussion is the Dalton's law which states, "The total pressure of a gas mixture is equal to the sum of the partial pressures of the component gases." To calculate the P of a particular gas, multiply the total pressure (P_T) of all the gases times the fraction of composition of the gas you are trying to find.

At sea level (1 atmosphere) the total gas pressure (P_T) is 760 mm Hg. Oxygen is approximately 20.93% of the total atmospheric composition. Therefore, the partial pressure of O_2 (PO_2) is:

$$760 \times 0.2093 = 159.1 \text{ mm Hg}$$
$$159.1 \text{ mm Hg} = \text{the approximate } PO_2 \text{ in atmospheric air}$$

The P_T of the two gases in the box equals 760 mm Hg (Figure 5-1). Gas (a) equals 2/10 or 20% of the P_T. Gas (b) equals 8/10 or 80% of the P_T. Therefore, the P of gas (a) is:

$$0.20 \times 760 = 152 \text{ mm Hg}$$

The P of gas (b) is:

$$0.80 \times 760 = 608 \text{ mm Hg}$$

The understanding of partial pressures, as they relate to respiratory physiology, requires a comparison of air composition between the atmospheric and the alveolar air. From Table 5-1, it can be seen that the total pressure of the atmospheric air and the alveolar air is the same.

However, when comparing the two, it is important to note the difference in the percentage and P of each of the component gases. Above any solution is the vapor of the solution (solvent) itself. This is known as the vapor pressure. Under equilibrium conditions, the P of a gas in a liquid is equal to the partial pressure of the gas above the liquid. The vapor pressure of water at 37°C is

TABLE 5-1 Understanding Partial Pressures				
Specific Gases		**Dry Atmosphere Air**		**Alveolar Air**
Nitrogen	N_2	79.03	600.60 mm Hg	74.9	569.24 mm Hg
Oxygen	O_2	20.93	159.10 mm Hg	13.6	103.36 mm Hg
Carbon dioxide	CO_2	0.04	0.30 mm Hg	5.3	40.28 mm Hg
Water	H_2O	-	-	6.2	47.12 mm Hg
Total		100.00	760.00 mm Hg	100.00	760.00 mm Hg

approximately 47 mm Hg. The airways of the lungs, including the alveoli, are fully saturated with water vapor, ie, 100% relative humidity. This means a partial pressure of water vapor within these airways equaling approximately 47 mm Hg. This water vapor pressure must appear as part of the total gas pressure and this is reflected by a decrease in the partial pressures of the other gases within the alveoli. Another gas law which may help explain the relationship of Ps above and within a solution is Henry's law which states, "The quantity of a gas that dissolves in a volume of liquid is directly proportional to the partial pressure of that gas, the pressure remaining constant."

Diffusion

It is within the alveoli that gas exchange takes place. The exchange of gases between the alveoli and the venous blood returning to the lungs is a result of the gases diffusing across the alveolar and capillary membranes. The ability of a gas to diffuse across these membranes and either into or out of the blood is dependent upon five factors. Certain pathologies such as COPD, pulmonary edema, tumors, and fibrosis, can all affect the efficiency of gas transfer. The factors affecting diffusion are:

1. The solubility of the gas in the fluid.
2. The concentration or pressure gradient.
3. The amount of surface area available.
4. The thickness of the membrane.
5. The temperature of the fluid.

Gases diffuse from an area of high concentration (pressure) to an area of low concentration (pressure) until equilibrium is attained. In this way, essential gases move into and out of the blood via the lungs.

Oxygen Dissociation

The way in which O_2 is taken up and given off can be seen graphically using an oxygen hemoglobin dissociation curve. The resulting S-shaped curve will show the percentage of saturated hemoglobin (left vertical axis) at varying partial pressures of oxygen (horizontal axis). Example of this curve is shown in Figure 5-2. At maximal saturation, each gram of hemoglobin has an oxygen carrying capacity of 1.34 mL/100 mL of blood (PO_2 = 760 mm Hg), or 4 O_2 molecules per hemoglobin. The average adult has between 14 and 16 g of hemoglobin for every 100 mL of blood. Venous blood has a PO_2 of 40 mm Hg at rest. This means that 75% of the hemoglobin is saturated in "deoxygenated" blood.

Factors Affecting Affinity of Oxygen for Hemoglobin

The three major factors which affect the affinity of oxygen for hemoglobin are blood acidity (pH), PCO_2, and temperature. The oxygen-hemoglobin dissociation curve (Figure 5-2) is affected by any one of these factors. The curve will shift either:

- Downward and to the right.
- Upward and to the left.

An increase in hydrogen ion concentration (lowering the pH) causes the blood to be more acidic which causes the curve to shift downward and to the right. When the curve shifts downward and to the right, as in an acidotic state,

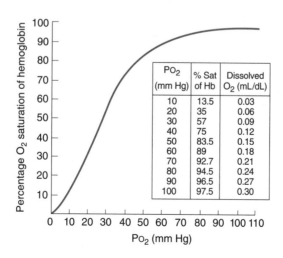

Figure 5-2 • Oxygen-hemoglobin dissociation curve.
Redrawn and reproduced with permission from Comroe JH Jr, et al. *The Lung: Clinical Physiology and Pulmonary Function Tests.* 2nd ed. Year Book, 1962.

O_2 doesn't bond as easily or as strongly at the level of the lungs; however O_2 is more readily released to the tissue levels. Increases in temperature also have a similar effect on the curve.

Conversely, a decrease in hydrogen ion concentration (increase in pH or alkalosis), a reduction in PCO_2, or lowering of the temperature will cause the curve to shift upward and to the left. This causes oxygen bind more readily and more tightly to hemoglobin at the level of the lungs, however, O_2 is not as readily released from hemoglobin at the tissue level.

Carbon Dioxide (Co₂) Transport

Carbon dioxide is a by-product of normal aerobic cellular metabolism. Under resting conditions, each 100 mL of blood gives up 4 to 5 mL of CO_2 in the lungs. Carbon dioxide is very acidic and is transported by the blood until it can be eliminated from the body by either the lungs or excreted by kidneys. Inability of the body to excrete CO_2 would result in the blood becoming too acidic to sustain life. Carbon dioxide is transported in the blood in three ways.

These are:

- Carried in the form of bicarbonate
- Combined with hemoglobin (carbaminohemoglobin)
- Dissolved in plasma

Although CO_2 is almost 20-fold more soluble than oxygen in plasma, only 7% to 10% is carried in this form. A larger amount (23%-25%) diffuses into the red blood cell (RBC) and combines with hemoglobin (Hb) to form carbamino-hemoglobin ($HbCO_2$).

$$Hb + CO_2 \rightarrow HbCO_2$$

The largest amount of carbon dioxide (65%-70%) is carried in the form of bicarbonate (HCO_3^-).

This reaction occurs quite slowly in plasma but upon entering the RBC the reaction is increased almost 1000-fold by the assistance of the enzyme carbonic anhydrase.

$$\overset{\text{Carbonic}}{CO_2 + H_2O \rightarrow H_2CO_3}$$
Anhydrase

Carbon dioxide combines with water to form carbonic acid. The carbonic acid (H_2CO_3) then dissociates into a hydrogen ion (H^+) and a HCO_3^-.

$$H_2CO_3 \rightarrow H^+ + HCO_3^-$$

The free H+s produced by this reaction are buffered primarily by deoxyhemoglobin. The HCO_3^-s formed diffuse into the plasma. As the bicarbonate ions move out of the cell chloride ions (Cl^-) move into the cell in a 1:1 relationship. This phenomenon is known as the chloride shift. It occurs so that electrochemical neutrality is maintained within the cell. In the lungs this chemical reaction reverses as CO_2 is expelled.

Oxygen Delivery Systems

The purpose of oxygen therapy is to:

1. Increase PO_2 in the alveoli and the blood.
2. Reduce the ventilatory workload.
3. Reduce the myocardial workload.

The major functions of both the cardiovascular and respiratory system are to supply oxygen to the tissues and remove metabolic waste. Reducing the workload causes a decrease in O_2 utilization and waste production. Once it has been decided that the patient would benefit from receiving supplemental oxygen, the correct oxygen-delivery device must be selected. Devices that deliver O_2 to the patient fall into four groups: low flow, conserving, high flow, and enclosures.

Low-flow device such as nasal cannulas, simple face masks and reservoir masks deliver oxygen at rates below the normal patient inspiratory flow rate of about 30 liters per minute (L/min). The patient draws in room air along with the supplemental oxygen. Nasal cannulas give more freedom than a mask and prevent patients from feeling claustrophobic using a mask and are a good choice for patients who are mouth breathers.

Conserving devices are designed to decrease the O_2 flow needed to provide adequate oxygenation. These devices can reduce oxygen requirements by at least 50%. For example, a patient who needs a flow of 3 L/min can reduce their flow to 1.5 L/min with a conserving device. Conserving devices include oxygen systems that require periodic refilling (cylinders or liquid oxygen systems).

High-flow devices deliver O_2 at rates above the normal inspiratory flow rate and maintain a fixed concentration of oxygen with inspiration regardless of the inspiratory flow and breathing pattern. One of the most commonly used device systems is the venture mask which uses a nozzle to accelerate the oxygen flow and mix the O_2 with air at a precise rate. A venture mask can easily deliver 24% to 50% of oxygen by using different adapters with different sized nozzle openings.

Enclosure devices are typically used for neonates and infants. These devices enclose the patient's head or whole body and provide an oxygen-enriched

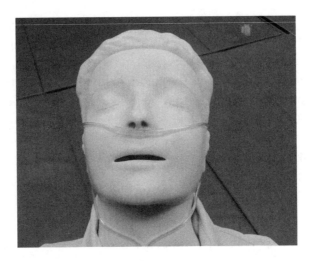

Figure 5-3 • Nasal prongs.

atmosphere to treat hypoxemia (condition where the body does not receive enough oxygen). A rigid clear plastic hood is filled with oxygen. A croup tent (cool mist tent) is an example of an enclosure device. It is a large clear plastic tent that covers a hospital crib and provides 22% to 40% oxygen and a cool mist to reduce upper airway edema.

Nasal Prongs

Nasal prongs (cannula) are effective in patients who do not require more than 30% to 40% oxygen (Figure 5-3). This device utilizes the patient's own anatomical reservoir of O_2 (found in the nasopharynx, oropharynx, and hypopharynx) which mixes with the room air entrained with each breath. Oxygen flow rates should never exceed 6 L/min as this would cause rapid drying and dehydration of the nasal mucosa. Flow rates more than 6 L/min will not cause a significant increase in fraction of inspired oxygen (FIO_2) and therefore result in a waste of O_2. Patients who will not tolerate a mask may accept nasal cannula, which may prove to be the only alternative even though a high FIO_2 cannot be obtained (Table 5-2).

Non-Rebreather (Reservoir) Mask

In contrast to the nasal cannula, the non-rebreather mask utilizes not only the anatomical reservoir but the mask and the reservoir bag that is attached to it (Figure 5-4). This device is intended to supply high concentrations of oxygen

TABLE 5-2 Oxygen Concentrations for the Nasal Cannula	
Flow rate	**Oxygen Concentration**
1	24%
2	28%
3	32%
4	36%
5	40%
6	44%

at FIO_2's between 60% and 95%. Examples where this device may be utilized include serious trauma, carbon monoxide poisoning, myocardial infarction, pulmonary edema, etc. Flow rates below 6 L/min should not be used as it may provide insufficient oxygen to fill the reservoir (Table 5-3).

Venturi Mask

Venturi masks are designed to provide a fixed concentration of oxygen (Figure 5-5). Selection of a prescribed oxygen concentration is provided via the use of the appropriate oxygen diluter jet available and adjusting the O_2 flow to the appropriate level. The oxygen flow to the mask cannot be humidified. Humidity is added to the mask separately through a special attachment.

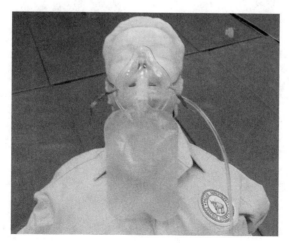

Figure 5-4 • Non-rebreather mask.

TABLE 5-3 Oxygen Concentrations for the Non-Rebreather Mask	
Flow Rate	**Oxygen Concentration (Estimated)**
6	60%
7	70%
8	80%
9	90%
10	95%+
12	95%+
15	95%+

Aerosol Mask

The aerosol mask is not something routinely used unless administering medications (Figure 5-6). The design of this mask is such that the O_2 entrained into it picks up sterile normal saline usually containing a medication, that is, albuterol. As the oxygen passes through the nebulizer it picks up molecular and particulate saline containing medication. This medication is then transferred to the patient via the respiratory system. At approximately 5 or 6 L/O_2 this device will provide an FIO_2 of about 40% oxygen.

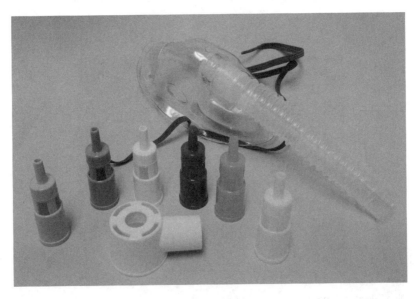

Figure 5-5 • Venturi mask.

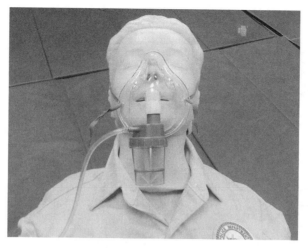

Figure 5-6 • Aerosol mask.

Bag-Valve Mask and Oxygen-Powered Ventilators

Both of these devices can supply 100% O_2 to a patient by either positive pressure or free flow oxygen (Figure 5-7). Primarily, they are used to ventilate patients who are either not breathing or have insufficient ventilatory function.

While both will do the job, the O_2-powered ventilators do not allow the operator a feel for the patient's lung compliance. Decreasing compliance is a significant clinical finding. The operator can also feel and hear whether the gas is being supplied to the lungs.

The O_2-powered systems deliver O_2 at a very rapid rate (around 1.6 L/sec) and commonly cause an increase in airway pressures. Although most are equipped with a pressure blow off at around 60 cm H_2O gastric distention is common. This is caused by the gastric sphincter muscle in the esophagus having a release point of around 40 cm H_2O. Therefore even with proper use,

TABLE 5-4 Oxygen Concentrations for the Venturi Mask		
Orange	50% oxygen	10 l.p.m.
Pink	40% oxygen	8 l.p.m.
Green	35% oxygen	8 l.p.m.
White	31% oxygen	6 l.p.m.
Yellow	28% oxygen	4 l.p.m.
Blue	24% oxygen	4 l.p.m.

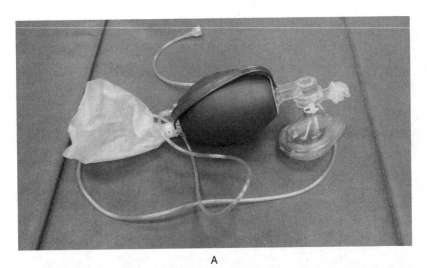

A

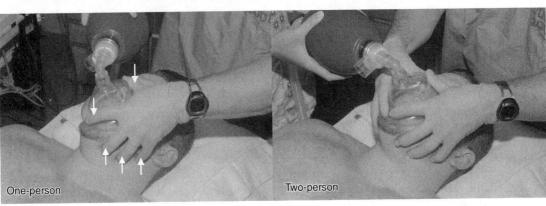

One-person

Two-person

B

Figure 5-7 • Bag-valve mask and oxygen-powered ventilators.
Reproduced with permission from Knoop KJ, Stack LB, Storrow AB, Thurman RJ, eds. *The Atlas of Emergency Medicine.*
3rd ed. (Photo Contributor: Lawrence B. Stack, MD.) Copyright © McGraw-Hill Education. All rights reserved.

dangerous and rapid gastric distention may occur causing a decrease in lung volume and an increase potential for vomiting.

The bag-valve mask system supplies 100% O_2 to the patient when connected to a 15 L/min O_2 source and the reservoir bag is attached. Should the reservoir bag not be used, approximately 60% O_2 can be delivered.

Bag-Valve Mask Ventilation Pearls

- It is crucial to know how to use this device properly
- C-shape over mouth (Figure 5-7b)

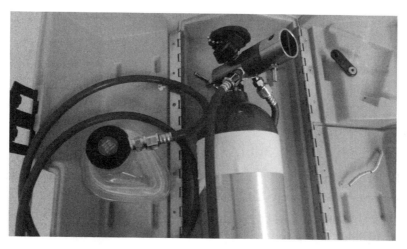

Figure 5-8 · Oxygen-powered ventilator.

- E-shape over mandible (keep fingers on mandible *not* soft tissues as this can occlude the airway) (Figure 5-7b)
- Can be difficult because small position changes can have big effect
- Can be difficult because kids will desaturate faster
- Mask size is a unique concern
- If you don't have a small mask, use a big one and turn it upside down
- Trouble bagging → two nasal airways, oral airway, then bag
- Vomiting during bagging → place an orogastric or nasogastric tube (OG or NG), empty stomach, continue bagging
- Self-inflating bag or manual inflating reservoir bags are both option
- Pop-off pressure valves generally go off at >40 cm H_2O; these should be manually disabled for ventilation of patients with higher airway pressures

KEY POINTS

Too much pressure is used in an attempt to make a seal and the airway is actually obstructed by the person doing the bagging ("white-knuckle" sign); proper technique should lift the jaw into the mask to (jaw thrust) create a seal.

Tidal Volumes

- Generally 10 to 15 mL/kg
- Clinically enough to get adequate chest expansions

- How big should the reservoir bag be?
  - Neonate: 250 mL
  - Infant: 500 mL
  - Children: 1 to 2 L
  - Adults: 3 to 5 L

Hazards and Complications of Oxygen Therapy

Although as common as the air we breathe, O_2 is also a drug that can be dangerous if used improperly. Various hazards and complications are associated with oxygen therapy. The use of oxygen poses a fire hazard as oxygen makes flammable items burn much faster and hotter. Never allow an open flame in the presence of O_2.

There are three complications related to the increased amounts of inspired oxygen.

- Oxygen induced hypoventilation or apnea (cessation of breathing). This mainly occurs with COPD patients (carbon dioxide retainers). These patients cannot expel all of the carbon dioxide out of their lungs. Supplementing oxygen given to these patients causes the oxygen levels to elevate potentially leading to a loss of drive to breathe resulting in the cessation of breathing.
- Absorption atelectasis, inhaling high levels of O_2 replaces the gasses in the alveoli reducing the gas volume. Oxygen is absorbed into the blood more quickly decreasing the residual volume, and preventing expansion in the alveoli.
- Oxygen toxicity (poisonous) occurs with prolonged or continuous high concentrations of supplemental oxygen.

Calculation of Tank Duration

To determine the duration or amount of oxygen in a gas cylinder, a formula may be used.

$$\text{Duration of flow (minutes)} = \frac{[\text{Gauge pressure (psi)} - \text{Safe residual pressure (SRP)}] \times \text{Constant of the tank}}{\text{Flow rate (L / min)}}$$

Constant Factor Tank Capacity Gauge Pressure (Full)

- D cylinder 0.16 350 L
- E cylinder 0.28 625 L
- M cylinder 1.56 3000 L

The safe residual pressure for all oxygen tanks is 200 psi.

What is the duration of tank M, when using a flow rate of 10 L/min?

$$\text{Duration of flow} = 2000 - 200 \times 1.56/10 = 2808$$
$$2808/10 = 281 \text{ minutes (4 h, 41 min)}$$

REVIEW QUESTIONS

1. _____ such as nasal cannulas, simple face masks and reservoir masks deliver oxygen at rates below the normal patient inspiratory flow rate of about 30 L/min. The patient draws in room air along with the supplemental oxygen.

   A. Conserving device
   B. High-flow device
   C. Low-flow device
   D. None of the above

   Correct answer is d.

2. You are treating a 76-year-old male patient in congestive heart failure. The patient has dyspnea and audible rales. He is 2/3 full from the bases to apices. As you are getting the CPAP device ready, you need to estimate how long you have before you need to change the tank. You are using a full E tank (2000 psi) and setting the flow at 15 (l p.m). Using the formula provided in this chapter, determine the duration or amount of oxygen you have in this gas cylinder.

   A. 45 min
   B. 23 min
   C. 34 min
   D. 10 min

   Correct answer is c.

3. Carbon dioxide is transported in the blood in three ways. These are:

   A. carried in the form of bicarbonate.
   B. combined with hemoglobin (carbaminohemoglobin).
   C. dissolved in plasma.
   D. all the above are correct.

   Correct answer is d.

4. **Typically, there are three complications related to the increased amounts of inspired oxygen.**

   A. Oxygen induced hypoventilation or apnea (cessation of breathing). This mainly occurs with COPD patients (carbon dioxide retainers).

   B. Flow rates higher than 6 L/min will not cause a significant increase in FIO_2 and therefore result in a waste of oxygen. Patients who will not tolerate a mask may accept nasal cannula, which may prove to be the only alternative even though a high FIO_2 cannot be obtained.

   C. Oxygen toxicity occurs with prolonged or continuous high concentrations of supplemental oxygen causing toxicity (poisonous).

   D. Answers a and c are correct.

Correct answer is d.

5. **High-flow devices deliver oxygen at rates above the normal inspiratory flow rate and maintain a fixed concentration of O_2 with inspiration regardless of the inspiratory flow and breathing pattern. One of the most commonly used device systems is the venture mask, which uses a nozzle to accelerate the oxygen flow and mix the oxygen with air at a precise rate. A venture mask can easily deliver 24% to 50% of O_2 by using different adapters with different sized nozzle openings.**

   A. True

   B. False

Correct answer is a.

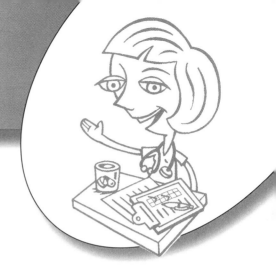

chapter 6

Respiratory Pharmacology

LEARNING OBJECTIVES

At the completion of this chapter, the learner will be able to:

1. Describe the pathophysiology of certain disease states and the rationale for the use of selected pharmacotherapy interventions.

2. Explain the pharmacology (mechanism of action, effects, pharmacokinetics, side effects, etc.) of the drugs discussed for each disease.

3. Discuss drugs of choice and alternatives for a given patient and disease.

4. Anticipate potential side effects, recognize adverse reactions, and discuss their management.

KEY TERMS

Acetylcholine

Alpha$_1$-agonists

Alpha$_2$-agonists

Anti-tussives

Autonomic nervous system

Beta agonists

Central nervous system

Dopamine

Epinephrine

Muscarinic

Neurotransmitters of the ANS

Norepinephrine

Parasympathetic

Sympathetic

Scenario

Your 76-year-old female patient has been a two-pack-a-day smoker since the age of 15, and has chronic bronchitis. She called you today because she has not felt well for about a week and says she is tired of fighting for every breath. You'll notice she is cyanotic, and has a productive cough. Her cardiorespiratory system relies on _____ as the main drive for respiration.

1. oxygen pressure (PaO$_2$)

2. alkalemia

3. carbon dioxide pressure (PaCO$_2$)

4. acidemia

Correct answer is 1. The hypoxic drive is a form of respiratory drive in which the body uses oxygen chemoreceptor's instead of carbon dioxide (CO$_2$) receptors to regulate the respiratory cycle. Normal respiration is driven mostly by the levels of CO$_2$ in the arteries, which are detected by peripheral chemoreceptors, and very little by the oxygen (O$_2$) levels. An increase in CO$_2$ will cause chemoreceptor reflexes to trigger an increase in respirations. Hypoxic drive accounts normally for 10% of the total drive to breathe. This increases as the PaO$_2$ goes to 70 torr and below, while hypoxic drive is no longer active when PaO$_2$ exceeds 170 torr. In the past, it was believed that in cases where there are chronically high CO$_2$ levels in the blood such as in chronic obstructive pulmonary disease (COPD) patients, the body will begin to rely more on the oxygen receptors and less on the carbon dioxide receptors. And that in this case, when there is an increase in O$_2$ levels the body will decrease the rate of respirations. Recent studies have proven that COPD patients who have chronically compensated elevated CO_2 levels (CO_2 retainers) are not in fact dependent on hypoxic drive to breathe. However, when in respiratory failure and put on high inspired O_2, the CO_2 in their blood may increase via three mechanisms, namely, the Haldane effect, the ventilation/perfusion mismatch (where the regional pulmonary hypoxic vasoconstriction is released), and by the removal or reduction of the hypoxic drive itself.

Introduction

To discuss the pharmacology of the sympathetic and parasympathetic nervous system can be overwhelming. The number of drugs that influence these systems is immense, and you will be hard-pressed to find drugs that do not either directly or indirectly interact with the sympathetic and parasympathetic nervous system. This chapter will discuss agonists and antagonists of the following receptors: α receptors, β receptors, dopamine receptors (sympathetic receptors), muscarinic (M) receptors, and nicotinic receptors. Again, this subject could become overwhelming, as each organ in the body expresses these receptors. Sometimes, the same receptor can have different responses for different organs.

Lungs

The two main actions of drugs affecting the lungs occur by:

1. affecting airway diameter.
2. affecting airway secretions.

The two receptors involved in this control are β_2 and M receptors.

1. Airway diameter: bronchodilation-sympathetic activity epinephrine
   - epinephrine (α_1, α_2, β_1, β_2)
   - exogenous β_2 agonists (albuterol and other similar drugs), which causes bronchial smooth muscle dilation and decreased secretions in the lungs. Withdrawal of these agents or decreased sympathetic activity causes bronchiolar relaxation, and increases bronchiolar secretions.
   - the antimuscarinic agent ipratropium bromide, a muscarinic-receptor antagonist, is very effective in blocking muscarinic bronchoconstriction and increased secretion. It is a quaternary amine; therefore it crosses membranes poorly and is excellent for inhalation and targeting to the lungs with minimal systemic side effects.

2. Epinephrine and dopamine can be used for emergencies where increased ventilation is required, but due to their systemic side effects, are not used for long-term therapy.

3. Norepinephrine has little effect on the lungs because of its specificity for α receptors.

4. Bronchoconstriction: Muscarinic-receptor activity results in decreased airway diameter with increased secretions. Muscarinic drugs are not used for this action, as there is little indication for decreasing the diameter of the airways. Specifically, we look for antimuscarinic agents that perform the opposite.

Anatomy of the Autonomic Nervous System

The central nervous system (CNS) receives varied internal and external stimulus. This stimulus is integrated and expressed subconsciously through the autonomic nervous system to adjust the involuntary functions of the body. The somatic nerves that innervate voluntary skeletal muscle are not part of the autonomic system.

The autonomic nervous system consists of two large divisions:

- Sympathetic (thoracolumbar) "Fight-or-Flight": The sympathetic nervous system is responsible for regulating many homeostatic mechanisms in living organisms. Fibers from the sympathetic nervous system innervate tissues in almost every organ system, providing at least some regulatory function to things as diverse as pupil diameter, gut motility, and urinary output. It is perhaps best known for mediating the neuronal and hormonal stress response commonly known as the "fight-or-flight" response. This response is also known as sympathoadrenal response of the body. This response acts primarily on the cardiovascular system, and is mediated directly via impulses transmitted through the sympathetic nervous system and indirectly via catecholamines secreted from the adrenal medulla.

- Parasympathetic (craniosacral) "Feed and Breed": The parasympathetic nervous system is a portion of the visceral (autonomic) branch of the peripheral nervous system (PNS). The regions of the body associated with this division are the cranial and sacral regions of the spinal cord. Specifically, cranial nerves III, VII, IX, X (vagus nerve) and in the sacral region (spinal nerves exiting from the sacrum) the spinal nerves S_2 to S_4. Because its cells begin as cranial nerves and exit in the sacral regions of the spine, the CNS is said to have a craniosacral outflow.

Similar to the sympathetic division, the parasympathetic division also has pre and postganglionic neurons. Typically, in the parasympathetic division the ganglion will be closer to the area of innervation—unlike the sympathetic ganglion which form immediately lateral and inferior to the spinal nerve—making up the so-called "chain ganglion." Both divisions are defined by their anatomic origin rather than by their physiological characteristics.

Neurotransmitters of the Autonomic Nervous System

- The primary neurochemical mediator of both sympathetic and parasympathetic preganglionic neurons is acetylcholine (ACh).
- The primary mediator of sympathetic postganglionic fibers is norepinephrine (NE), but at least some sympathetic postganglionic fibers to sweat glands are cholinergic (ACh).
- The mediators of parasympathetic postganglionic fibers are ACh.
- Epinephrine is found in the adrenal medulla, the CNS, and the paraaortic bodies.
- Dopamine is a neurochemical mediator in the CNS and probably also in some neurons in the superior cervical ganglion and the kidneys.
- Norepinephrine, epinephrine, and dopamine are sometimes collectively referred to as catecholamines.
- Drugs that resemble catecholamines functionally and structurally are also called sympathomimetic amines.

Metabolism of Acetylcholine

- Acetylcholine (ACh) is synthesized by choline acetyl-transferase, a soluble cytoplasmic enzyme that catalyzes the transfer of an acetyl group from acetyl-coenzyme A to choline.
- The activity of choline acetyl-transferase is much greater than the maximal rate at which ACh synthesis occurs. Choline acetyl-transferase inhibitors have little effect to alter the level of this bound ACh. ACh is stored in a bound form in vesicles. Choline must be pumped into the cholinergic neuron, and the action of the choline transporter is the rate-limiting step in ACh synthesis.
- Upon the arrival of an action potential in the cholinergic neuron terminal, voltage sensitive calcium channels open and ACh stores are released by exocytosis to trigger a postsynaptic physiological response.

- This action is terminated by the rapid hydrolysis of ACh into choline and acetic acid, a reaction catalyzed by the enzyme acetylcholinesterase. The transient, discrete, localized action of ACh is due in part to the great velocity of this hydrolysis. The choline liberated locally by acetylcholinesterase can be reutilized by presynaptic reuptake and resynthesis into ACh.

What Went Wrong?

Pralidoxime is an antidote to organophosphate pesticides and chemicals. Organophosphates bind to the esteratic site of acetylcholinesterase, which results initially in reversible inactivation of the enzyme. Acetylcholinesterase inhibition causes acetylcholine to accumulate in synapses, producing continuous stimulation of cholinergic fibers throughout the nervous systems. If given within 24 hours after organophosphate exposure, pralidoxime reactivates the acetylcholinesterase by cleaving the phosphate-ester bond formed between the organophosphate and acetylcholinesterase.

In addition to acetylcholinesterase which is found near cholinergic neurons and in red blood cells (but not in plasma), there is also a nonspecific cholinesterase which is present in plasma and in some organs but not in the red blood cell (RBC) or the cholinergic neuron.

Norepinephrine and Epinephrine

The actions of α and β adrenoreceptors are mediated by various intracellular mechanisms. Activation of β adrenoreceptors by neurotransmitter, hormone, or drug leads to synthesis of cyclic adenosine monophosphate (cAMP) by adenylyl cyclase at the cytoplasmic facet of the plasma membrane. For the purposes of simplicity we use the following classification scheme (see Figures 6-1 and 6-2):

1. α_1, α_2
2. $\beta_1, \beta_2, \beta_3$

Alpha$_1$-Agonists

An adrenergic α-agonist is a drug which selectively stimulates α-adrenergic receptors. The α-adrenergic receptor has two subclasses: α_1 and α_2. Although complete selectivity between receptors is rarely achieved, phenylephrine is an α_1 agonist and clonidine is a α_2 partial agonist. The dilator muscle of the pupil is constricted giving mydriasis (dilated pupil). Some of the smooth muscle tissue in the eyelids is constricted leading to a widened palpebral fissure. Most arterioles are constricted and peripheral vascular resistance is increased, raising blood pressure. Veins are also constricted leading to a central

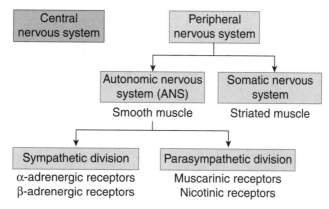

FIGURE 6-1 • Peripheral nervous system.
Reproduced with permission from Hoffman BL, Schorge JO, Schaffer JI, Halvorson LM, Bradshaw KD, Cunningham FG, Calver LE, eds. *Williams Gynecology*. 2nd ed. 2012. New York: Copyright © McGraw-Hill Education. All rights reserved.

redistribution of blood into the thorax. Stimulation of pilomotor nerves causes hair to "stand on end" (piloerection). The associated stimulation of myoepithelial tissue in the vicinity of the apocrine glands (axilla, crural areas) causes gland emptying although the glands themselves are not stimulated. Bladder sphincters are contracted by α_1-stimulation. The spleen capsule is contracted. There is CNS stimulation with agents which cross the blood-brain barrier (Norepinephrine, dopamine, and epinephrine do not). Some agonists at α_1-adrenoreceptors increase myocardial contractility (but not heart rate) in some circumstances, but α_1 stimulation of contractility is more important clinically. Norepinephrine is very close to phenylephrine in its effects and has enjoyed wider clinical use in the treatment of shock. Norepinephrine differs from phenylephrine primarily in having a greater capacity to stimulate α_1 adrenoreceptors as well as α_1 adreno receptors. Epinephrine is used clinically primarily to support blood pressure, especially during anaphylaxis. Dopamine, the immediate metabolic precursor of norepinephrine, has wide use in the drug treatment of shock. At high but not at low dosages, it stimulates α_1 adrenoreceptors.

Alpha$_2$-Agonists

In many tissues pre-synaptic α_2 stimulation mediates feedback inhibition of norepinephrine release. When there is sufficient norepinephrine in the synaptic cleft to affect a response, it would be uneconomical of the neuron to continue to release still more transmitter.

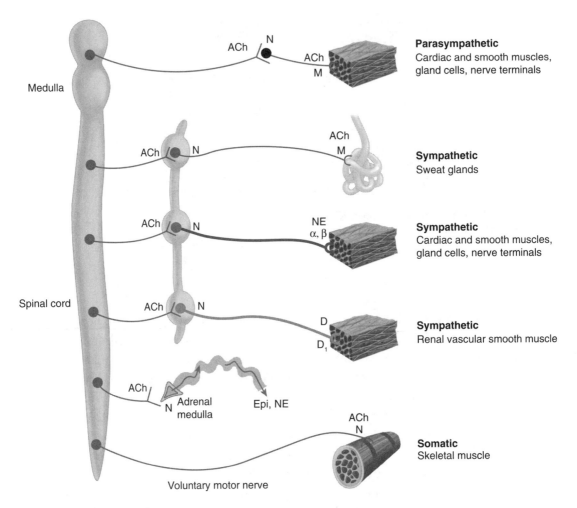

FIGURE 6-2 • Peripheral nervous system muscle innervation.
Reproduced with permission from Katzung BG, et al. *Basic and Clinical Pharmacology.* 11th ed. 2009. New York:
Copyright © McGraw-Hill Education. All rights reserved.

Beta Agonists

The drug isoproterenol stimulates both β_1- and β_2-receptors. The heart contracts with greater force (increased contractility) and heart rate is increased. Cardiac output rises. There is an increased likelihood of premature heartbeats and other arrhythmias. Arterioles are dilated, with resulting reduced resistance. Mean blood pressure is at least transiently lowered. A gravid uterus is relaxed. Bronchioles are relaxed (useful in asthmatics) and metabolic effects on the liver and adipose tissue lead to hyperglycemia and lipolysis. Some CNS stimulation occurs. While it is advantageous to stimulate β_2 receptors in the bronchial tree of asthmatic patients or the uterus of a woman in premature labor, the β_1-cardiac stimulation is an unwanted effect. This has led to efforts to achieve selective β_2 stimulation. A variety of recognized β_2-agonists have been developed, but their selectivity is partial. In certain patients, the cardiac stimulation of β-agonists is desirable (pulmonary edema, coronary bypass post-op) and a relatively selective β_1 agonist such as dobutamine is indicated. Moderate doses of dobutamine increase myocardial contractility without significantly altering blood pressure. The relatively small effect of dobutamine on blood pressure is due to counter-balancing effects of β_1 stimulation and β_2 stimulation on arteriolar and venous tone.

A β_3 adrenoreceptor has been identified and is sensitive to norepinephrine and not easily blocked by the usual β antagonists. It mediates thermogenesis in skeletal muscle and energy expenditure in adipose tissue.

Impairment of respiratory function due to viral or bacterial infection, asthma, or COPD has a major impact on the health of a patient. We will examine the various classes of drugs used to treat respiratory dysfunction. In particular, this section focuses on:

1. Anti-tussives and expectorants used in the treatment of cough
2. Agents used as decongestants
3. Agents used in the treatment of asthma
4. Agents used in the treatment of COPD

Relief of Cough

There are two types of cough. These are:

- Productive: leads to removal of sputum from the lungs
- Dry cough: no removal of sputum

Treatment of cough mainly consists of treating the underlying cause. A productive cough should not be suppressed except in special circumstances (ie, when it exhausts the patient or prevents rest and sleep) and generally not until the cause has been identified. Suppressing a productive cough is less advisable because sputum needs to be cleared. Cough remedies are categorized as anti-tussives and expectorants.

Anti-tussives: Are either centrally or peripherally acting. Centrally acting anti-tussives inhibit or suppress the cough reflex by depressing the medullary cough center or associated higher centers. The most commonly used drugs in this group are dextromethorphan and codeine.

- Dextromethorphan (DXM), a congener of the narcotic analgesic levor-phanol, has no significant analgesic or sedative properties, does not depress respiration in usual doses, and is nonaddictive. No evidence of tolerance has been found during long-term use. Extremely high doses may depress respirations.

What Went Wrong?

Dextromethorphan (DXM), a common active ingredient found in many over-the-counter cough suppressant cold medicines, is used as a recreational drug for its dissociative effects. It has almost no psychoactive effects at medically recommended doses.

Dextromethorphan has powerful dissociative properties when adminis-tered in doses well above those considered therapeutic for cough suppres-sion. Recreational use of DXM is sometimes referred to in slang form as robo-tripping, whose prefix derives from the Robitussin brand name, or Triple Cs, which derives from the Coricidin brand (the pills were printed with "CCC").

- Codeine, which has anti-tussive, analgesic, and slight sedative effect, is especially useful in relieving a painful cough. It also exerts a drying action on the respiratory mucosa that may be useful (ie, in bronchorrhea) or deleterious (ie, when bronchial secretions are already viscous). At doses used for cough suppression, codeine has minimal respiratory depressant effects. Nausea, vomiting, constipation, tolerance to anti-tussive as well as analgesic effects, and physical dependence can occur, but potential for abuse is low.

Peripherally acting anti-tussives may act on either the afferent or the effer-ent side of the cough reflex. On the afferent side, an anti-tussive may reduce the input of stimuli by acting as a mild analgesic or anesthetic on the respira-tory mucosa; by modifying the output and viscosity of the respiratory tract fluid; or by relaxing the smooth muscle of the bronchi in the presence of bron-chospasm. On the efferent side, an anti-tussive may make secretions easier to cough up by increasing the efficiency of the cough mechanism. Peripherally acting agents are grouped as demulcents, and humidifying aerosols and steam inhalations.

- Demulcents are useful for coughs originating above the larynx. They form a protective coating over the irritated pharyngeal mucosa. They are usually given as syrups or lozenges and include acacia, licorice, glycerin, honey, and wild cherry syrups.

- Humidifying aerosols and steam inhalations exert an anti-tussive effect by acting as a demulcent and by decreasing the viscosity of bronchial secretions. Inhaling water as an aerosol or as steam, with or without medicaments (such as, sodium chloride, compound benzoin tincture, eucalyptol).

- Expectorants: These drugs help expel bronchial secretions from the respiratory tract by decreasing their viscosity. Expectorants facilitate removal by increasing the amount of respiratory tract fluid and exerting a demulcent action on the mucosal lining. Most expectorants increase secretions through reflex irritation of the bronchial mucosa. Some, such as the iodides, also act directly on the bronchial secretory cells and are excreted into the respiratory tract.

The use of expectorants is controversial. No objective experimental data show that any of the available expectorants decreases sputum viscosity or eases expectoration. Data may be lacking partly because of inadequate technology for obtaining such evidence. The use and choice of expectorants are often based on tradition and the widespread clinical impression that they are effective in some circumstances. Adequate hydration is the single most important measure that can be taken to encourage expectoration. If it is unsuccessful, using an expectorant in addition may produce the desired result. Iodides are used to liquefy tenacious bronchial secretions (ie, in late stages of bronchitis, bronchiectasis, and asthma). A saturated solution of potassium iodide is the least expensive, most commonly used preparation. Their usefulness is limited by low patient acceptance because they have an unpleasant taste and because side effects are common. The side effects are reversible and subside when the drug is stopped. Iodinated glycerol is better tolerated than potassium iodide solution but is probably less effective. Prolonged patient use of iodides or iodinated glycerol can lead to hypothyroidism.

- Guaifenesin is the most commonly used expectorant in OTC cough remedies. It has no serious adverse effects, but there is no clear evidence of its efficacy. Many other traditional expectorants are found in numerous Over-the-counter (OTC) cough remedies. Their efficacy is doubtful, particularly in the dosages of most preparations.

Less commonly used drugs: Mucolytics (ie, acetylcysteine) have free sulfhydryl groups that open mucoprotein disulfide bonds, reducing the viscosity of mucus. As a rule, their usefulness is restricted to a few special instances such as liquefying thick, tenacious, mucopurulent secretions (eg, in chronic bronchitis and cystic fibrosis). Acetylcysteine is given as a 10% to 20%

solution by nebulization or instillation. In some patients, mucolytics may aggravate airway obstruction by causing bronchospasm. If this occurs, these patients may inhale a nebulized sympathomimetic bronchodilator or take a formulation containing acetylcysteine (10%) and isoproterenol (0.05%) before taking the mucolytic.

- Decongestants: These agents are all adrenergic agonists. They exert their action by vasoconstriction of nasal blood vessels, reducing the volume of the nasal mucosa and opening up the airways. They can either be used topically for short-term relief or systemically for prolonged relief.
- Short-acting (topical) decongestants: Delivered as nasal sprays, these agents have the benefit of avoiding deleterious side-effects of systemic introduction of β agonists. The most commonly used short-acting agonist decongestant is phenylephrine. Repeated topical use of these compounds can lead to down-regulation of the receptors, and subsequent rebound hyperemia in the nasal blood vessels.
- Long-acting systemic decongestants: Used for prolonged duration of action, with an increased potential for systemic side effects. Pseudoephedrine is the most commonly used long-acting β agonist decongestant. Other agents such as ephedrine and phenylpropanolamine were formerly used, but they have been withdrawn from the OTC market.

Physiology of Asthma

Asthma is a chronic condition involving the respiratory system in which the airways occasionally constrict, become inflamed, and is lined with excessive amounts of mucus, often in response to one or more triggers. These episodes may be triggered by such things as exposure to an environmental stimulant such as an allergen, environmental tobacco smoke, cold or warm air, perfume, moist air, exercise or exertion, or emotional stress. In children, the most common triggers are viral illnesses such as those that cause the common cold. This airway narrowing causes symptoms such as wheezing, shortness of breath, chest tightness, and coughing. The airway constriction typically responds to bronchodilators. Between episodes, most patients feel well but can have mild symptoms and they may remain short of breath after exercise for longer periods of time than the normal individual. The symptoms of asthma, which can range from mild to life threatening, can usually, be controlled with a combination of drugs and environmental changes.

- Pathophysiology of asthma: Clinically characterized by recurrent, episodic bouts of coughing, wheezing, and shortness of breath.
- Quantitated by a reduction in forced expiratory volume in 1-second (FEV_1)
- Physiologically characterized by increased responsiveness of trachea and bronchi to various stimuli and by widespread narrowing that changes either spontaneously or in response to therapy.
- Pathologically characterized by contraction of airway smooth muscle, mucosal thickening from edema, and cellular infiltration.

Pathogenesis of Asthma

- Essentially a hyper-responsiveness to a number of substances that results in a reduction in the respiratory system's ability to provide sufficient airflow.
- Mediated by immunoglobulin E (IgE) antibodies bound to mast cells in airway mucosa.
- Re-exposure to antigen (pollen, fur, etc.), antigen-antibody reaction triggers the release of mediators stored in mast cell granules, and synthesis and release of other mediators.
- Early mediators include:
  - histamine
  - tryptase and other neutral proteases
  - leukotrienes (LTC4, LTD4)
  - prostaglandins
- Result of mediators is airway smooth muscle contraction and vascular leakage.
- Late mediators include:
  - granulocyte-macrophage colony stimulating factor (GM-CSF)
  - interleukins (IL4, IL5)
  - late mediators attract and activate eosinophil's and stimulate IgE production.
  - released mediators also activate neural pathways that can result in the release of compounds such as ACh at smooth muscle by vagal efferents resulting in contraction.

Therapeutic Approach to Asthma

- Asthmatic bronchospasm results from a combination of mediators released and an exaggerated response to their effects from the various steps involved in the process, there are several points of attack:
  - prevent mast cell degranulation
  - reducing bronchial responsiveness
  - relax airway smooth muscle

Cromolyn and Nedocromil

- Act by inhibiting mast cell degranulation, presumably by inhibiting delayed chloride channels, which are involved in the process of mast cell activation
- Effective only when used prophylactically
- Cannot reverse bronchospasm or alter bronchial tone
- Poorly absorbed from the gut, so delivered topically by inhalation of a microfine powder or aerosolized solution
- Can also be used as a nasal spray to reduce symptoms of allergic rhinitis
- Very few side effects, presumably due in part to the localized application of the drugs

Methylxanthines

- Act by reducing the breakdown of cAMP through the inhibition of phosphodiesterases.
- cAMP has bronchodilator activity through increasing the rate in inactivation of myosin light chain kinase (MLCK), an important component in smooth muscle contraction.
- Agents that elevate cAMP will lead to bronchodilation
- Methylxanthines taken orally can lead to a number of side effects due to increases in cAMP in a number of other systems:
  - CNS; nervousness and tremor
  - cardiovascular: positive chronotropic and inotropic effects
  - GI: stimulate secretion of gastric acid and digestive enzymes
  - renal: diuretic activity
  - need to measure plasma levels of these compounds in order to ensure that levels remain in the therapeutic range (5-20 mg/L for theophylline); toxicity is most common at levels > 20 mg/L.

Sympathomimetic Agents

- Beta-adrenergic receptor agonists, especially β_2 selective
- Work by elevating cAMP levels to promote bronchodilation.
- β_2-selective agonists do not have the chronotropic or inotropic effects of non selective or β_1-selective agonists.
- Non selective agents such as epinephrine, ephedrine, and isoproterenol are no longer or rarely used due to potential side effects.
- β_2-selective agonists are generally delivered either via metered-dose inhalers or nebulizer.

Commonly used medications include:

- Albuterol (Ventolin)®
- Metaproterenol (Alupent)®
- Terbutaline (Brethine)®
- Pirbuterol (Maxair)®
- Salmeterol (Servent)® is a long-acting β_2 agonist (12 hours or more). Thought to get its long-acting effect through the high lipid solubility of the compound, creating a "slow-release" depot within the airways.

Muscarinic Antagonists

- Inhibit effects of vagal-released acetylcholine at muscarinic receptors in the airways.
- Atropine is the classic muscarinic antagonist, but is not used due to systemic adverse effects.
- Ipratropium bromide can be delivered via inhaler and is poorly absorbed, resulting in few systemic effects.
- Takes up to 45 minutes to exert its effects, but effects can last for hours.

Corticosteroids have anti-inflammatory action which reduces the responsiveness of the airway. They do not reverse bronchospasm, but are thought to work mainly via inhibition of the production of cytokines.

- Can be delivered either orally, inhaled, or injected via IV or IM.
- Corticosteroids such as prednisone are usually only used in cases where urgent treatment is needed due to the problems with systemic actions of these agents such as adrenal suppression.
- Treatment with oral corticosteroids is usually for a fixed period (only 7 to 10 days).

- Dosages are usually reduced over the period of treatment to avoid rebound phenomena associated with drop in steroid levels.
- Inhaled steroids avoid these systemic effects, allowing them to be used in chronic/prophylactic treatment.
- Corticosteroid agents include:
  - beclomethasone (Beclovent, Vanceril)®
  - triamcinolone (Azmacort)®
  - fluticasone (Flovent)®

Leukotriene Pathway Inhibitors (Long-Term Asthma Care)

- Leukotrienes (in particular LTC4 and LTD4) are involved in the inflammatory response, so blocking their production or action can be a useful form of treatment.
- Leukotrienes are synthesized from arachidonic acid via 5-lipoxygenase, and bind to receptors on target tissues.
- Blocking production with 5-lipoxygenase inhibitors has been shown to be effective in both blocking response to antigen challenge. Currently used orally active compounds include zileuton (Zyflo).
  - Blocking actions of LTD4 at its receptor also reduces inflammatory response. Currently used orally active compounds include zafirlukast (Accolate).

Physiology of Chronic Obstructive Pulmonary Disease

Chronic obstructive pulmonary disease (COPD), also known as chronic obstructive airway disease (COAD), is a group of diseases characterized by the pathological limitation of airflow in the airway that is not fully reversible. It refers to an obstruction of airflow, which results in air becoming trapped in the lungs. COPD is the umbrella term for chronic bronchitis, emphysema, and a range of other lung disorders. It is most often caused by tobacco smoking, but can be due to other airborne irritants such as solvents as well as congenital conditions such as alpha-1 antitrypsin deficiency (AAT). According to the U.S. Department of Health and Human Services National Vital Statistics 2011 Report, ranks COPD as the third leading cause of death in the United States.

What Went Wrong?

Alpha-1 antitrypsin deficiency is a condition in which the body does not make enough of a protein that protects the lungs and liver from damage. The condition can lead to emphysema and liver disease.

Signs/Symptoms

- Shortness of breath with/or without exertion
- Other symptoms of COPD
- Symptoms of liver disease
- Unintentional weight loss
- Wheezing

Manifests as one of three pathological entities:

1. Chronic bronchitis
2. Chronic obstructive bronchitis
3. Emphysema

No drug treatment can affect the natural history of COPD. Treatment is designed toward correction of symptoms, maintenance of lung function, and improvement of quality of life.

- Since obstruction to airflow is the most typical characteristic of COPD, bronchodilators are drugs of first choice.
- In mild forms of COPD, a short-acting β_2 agonist such as albuterol followed by the muscarinic antagonist ipratropium are used on as "as needed" basis or before exercise.
- For more severe cases, short-acting β_2 agonists with ipratropium are prescribed on a regular basis (3-4 times per day).
- Theophylline is used when β agonists and ipratropium are ineffective; however, due to systemic effects of theophylline its use is declining.
- The efficacy of corticosteroids in the treatment of COPD is still under debate, but recent evidence suggests that inhaled corticosteroids, either alone or in combination with salmeterol, can result in a significant increase in FEV_1 in COPD patients. Chronic use of oral or systemic corticosteroids should be avoided.
- Leukotriene-synthesis inhibitors or leukotriene-receptor antagonists have not been adequately tested in COPD patients, so their use cannot be recommended at present.

Emergency Pharmacology

Albuterol (Proventil, Ventolin)®

Class   Relatively selective β_2-adrenergic bronchodilator.

Description   Albuterol is a sympathomimetic that is selective for β_2-adrenergic receptors. It relaxes smooth muscles of the bronchial tree and peripheral vasculature by stimulating adrenergic receptors of the sympathetic nervous system.

Onset and Duration   Onset: 5 to15 minutes after inhalation; 30 minutes Per Os (PO)

Duration: 3 to 4 hours after inhalation; 4 to 6 hours PO

Indications

- Relief of bronchospasm in patients with reversible obstructive airway disease.
- Prevention of exercise-induced bronchospasm.

Contraindications

- Prior hypersensitivity reaction to albuterol.
- Cardiac dysrhythmias associated with tachycardia.
- Tachycardia caused by digitalis intoxication

Adverse Reactions

- Tachycardia
- Restlessness
- Apprehension
- Headache
- Dizziness
- Nausea
- Palpitations
- Increase in blood pressure
- Dysrhythmias
- Hypokalemia

Drug Interactions   Sympathomimetics may exacerbate adverse cardiovascular effects. Antidepressants may potentiate the effects on the vasculature. Beta blockers may antagonize albuterol. Albuterol may potentiate diuretic-induced hypokalemia.

Dosage and Administration   Bronchial asthma

Adult: Albuterol sulfate solution 0.083% (one unit dose bottle of 3.0 mL), nebulized, at a flow rate that will deliver the solution over 5 to 15 minutes.

Pediatric: Albuterol sulfate 0.083% (one unit dose bottle of 3.0 mL), nebulized, at a flow rate that will deliver the solution over 5 to 15 minutes.

Aminophylline (Theophylline)®

Class   Xanthine bronchodilator

Actions   Smooth muscle relaxant, causes bronchodilation, has mild diuretic properties and increases heart rate.

Indications   Bronchial asthma, reversible bronchospasm associated with chronic bronchitis and emphysema, congestive heart failure, and pulmonary edema.

Contraindications   Patients with history of hypersensitivity to the drug, hypotension, patients with peptic ulcer disease.

Precautions   Monitor for arrhythmias. Monitor blood pressure. Do not administer to patients on chronic theophylline.

Side Effects   Convulsions, tremor, anxiety, dizziness, vomiting, palpitations, PVCs, and tachycardia.

Dosages   Method 1: 250 to 500 mg in 90 or 80 mL of D_5W, respectively, infused over 20 to 30 minutes (approximately 5-10 mg/kg/h)

Method 2: 250 to 500 mg (5-7 mg/kg) in 20 mL of D_5W infused over 20 to 30 minutes.

Routes   Slow IV infusion.

Pediatric Dosage   6 mg/kg loading dose to be infused over 20 to 30 minutes; maximum dose not to exceed 12 mg/kg per 24 hours.

Dexamethasone (Decadron, Hexadrol)®

Class   Steroid

Actions   May decrease cerebral edema, is an anti-inflammatory, and suppresses immune response (especially in allergic reactions).

Indications   Cerebral edema, anaphylaxis (after epinephrine and diphenhydramine), asthma, and COPD.

Contraindications   None in the emergency setting.

Precautions   Should be protected from heat, onset of action may be 2 to 6 hours and thus should not be considered to be of use in the critical first hour following an anaphylactic reaction.

Side Effects   Gastrointestinal bleeding and prolonged wound healing.

Dosage: 4 to 24 mg.

Pediatric Dosage: 0.2-0.5 mg/kg

Routes   IV

Diphenhydramine (Benadryl)®

Class   Antihistamine

Description   Antihistamines prevent the physiological actions of histamine by preventing histamine from reaching H_1- and H_2-receptor sites. Diphenhydramine also has anticholinergic (drying) and sedative effects. Antihistamines provide short-lived benefits and provide only symptomatic relief. Antihistamine is specific for conditions in which histamine excess is present (for example, acute urticaria) but is adjunctive therapy in the treatment of anaphylactic shock because epinephrine is more effective. Antihistamines are quite specific for reversing extrapyramidal reactions and are probably efficacious as drying agents in upper respiratory and sinus conditions.

Onset and Duration   Onset: Maximal affects 1 to 3 hours
    Duration: 6 to 12 hours

Indications

- Symptomatic relief of allergies
- Allergic reactions
- Anaphylaxis
- Acute dystonic reactions
- Motion sickness
- Antiparkinsonism

Contraindications

- Lower respiratory diseases such as asthma attacks
- Newborn or premature infants
- Nursing mothers
- Hypersensitivity
- Narrow angle glaucoma

Adverse Reactions

- Dose-related drowsiness
- Sedation
- Disrupted coordination
- Hypotension
- Palpitations
- Tachycardia
- Bradycardia
- Thickening of bronchial secretions

- Dry mouth and throat

- Epigastric distress

Drug Interactions   Central nervous system depressants and alcohol may have additive effects.

Monoamine oxidase inhibitors (MAO) inhibitors may prolong and intensify anticholinergic effects of antihistamines.

Dosage and Administration   50 mg, IV/saline lock bolus, or IM

Special Considerations   Pregnancy safety: Category B

Epinephrine (ADRENALIN)®

Class   Sympathomimetic

Description   Epinephrine stimulates α, β_1-, and β_2-adrenergic receptors in dose-related fashion. It is the initial drug of choice for treating bronchoconstriction and hypotension resulting from anaphylaxis as well as all forms of cardiac arrest. It is useful in managing reactive airway disease, but beta-adrenergic agents are often used initially because of their bronchial specificity and oral inhalation route. Rapid injection produces a rapid increase in systolic pressure, ventricular contractility, and heart rate. In addition, epinephrine causes vasoconstriction in the arterioles of the skin, mucosa, and splenic areas and antagonizes the effects of histamine.

Onset and Duration   Onset: (IM) 5 to 10 minutes; (IV) 1 to 2 minutes.

Duration: 5 to 10 minutes.

Indications

- Bronchial asthma

- Acute allergic reaction

- Cardiac arrest

- Asystole

- Pulseless electrical activity

- Ventricular fibrillation unresponsive to initial defibrillation attempts

Contraindications

- Hypersensitivity

- Hypovolemic shock

- Narrow angle glaucoma

Adverse Reactions

- Headache

- Nausea

- Restlessness
- Weakness
- Dysrhythmias
- Hypertension
- Precipitation of angina pectoris

Drug Interactions   MAO inhibitors and bretylium may potentiate the effect of epinephrine.

Beta-adrenergic antagonists may blunt inotropic response. Sympathomimetics and phosphodiesterase inhibitors may exacerbate dysrhythmia response. May be deactivated by alkaline solutions such as sodium bicarbonate and furosemide.

Dosage and Administration   **Asthma**

Epinephrine 0.3 mg (0.3 mL of a 1:1,000 solution), subcutaneously/intramuscular.

Anaphylactic Reaction   Epinephrine 1.0 mg (10 mL of a 1:10,000 solution), via the endotracheal (ET) tube. If endotracheal intubation has not been accomplished, administer epinephrine 0.3 mg (0.3 mL of a 1:1,000 solution), subcutaneously/intramuscular. Epinephrine 1.0 μg per minute, IV/saline lock drip. Prepare infusion by adding 1.0 mg of epinephrine (1.0 mL of a 1:1,000 solution) to 250 mL of normal saline (0.9) (1 μg per minute = 15 mL per hour = 15 gtt per minute). If there is insufficient improvement in hemodynamic status, the infusion may be increased until the desired therapeutic effects are achieved or adverse effects appear. (Maximum dosage is 4.0 μg per minute, IV/saline lock drip.)

Pediatric   **Anaphylactic reaction and newborn resuscitation:** Epinephrine 0.1 mg/kg (0.1 mL/kg of a 1:1,000 solution), IV/saline lock, IO, or ET.

Asthma   In patients of 1 year of age or older with severe respiratory distress, respiratory failure, and/or decreased breath sounds, administer epinephrine 0.01 mg/kg (0.01 mL/kg of a 1:1,000 solution), subcutaneously/intramuscular. Maximum dose is 0.3 mL.

Special Considerations   Pregnancy safety: Category C.

Syncope has occurred after epinephrine administration to asthmatic children. Epinephrine can increase myocardial oxygen demand.

Ipratropium bromide (Atrovent)®

Class   Anticholinergic.

Actions   Causes bronchodilation and dries respiratory tract secretions.

Indications   Bronchial asthma, reversible bronchospasm associated with chronic bronchitis and emphysema.

Contraindications   Patients with history of hypersensitivity to the drug should not be used as primary agent in acute treatment of bronchospasm.

Precautions   Blood pressure, pulse, and ECG must be constantly monitored.

Side Effects   Palpitations, dizziness, anxiety, tremors, headache, nervousness, dry mouth.

Dosage   Small-volume nebulizer: 500 µg should be placed in small volume nebulizer (typically administered with a β agonist).

Pediatric Dosage   Safety in children has not been established.

Routes   Inhalation only.

Isoetharine (Bronkosol)®

Class   Sympathomimetic (β_2 selective).

Actions   Bronchodilation

Indications   Asthma, reversible bronchospasm associated with chronic bronchitis and emphysema.

Contraindications   Patients with history of hypersensitivity to the drug.

Precautions   Blood pressure, pulse, and ECG must be constantly monitored.

Side Effects   Palpitations, tachycardia, anxiety and tremors, headache.

Dosage   Small-volume nebulizer: 0.5 mL (1:3 with saline).

Pediatric Dosage   0.25 to 0.5 mL diluted with 4 mL normal saline.

Routes   Inhalation only.

Magnesium Sulfate

Class   Electrolyte, CNS depressant

Description   Magnesium sulfate reduces striated muscle contractions and blocks peripheral neuromuscular transmission by reducing acetylcholine release at the myoneural junction. In emergency care, magnesium sulfate is used to manage seizures associated with toxemia of pregnancy. Other uses include uterine relaxation (to inhibit contractions of premature labor), as a bronchodilator after beta-agonist and anticholinergic agents have been used, replacement therapy for magnesium deficiency, as a cathartic to reduce the absorption of poisons from the GI tract, and in the initial therapy for convulsions.

Magnesium sulfate is gaining popularity as an initial treatment in the management of various dysrhythmias, particularly torsades de pointes, and dysrhythmias secondary to tricyclic antidepressant overdose or digitalis toxicity. The drug is also considered as a Class IIa agent (probably helpful) for refractory ventricular fibrillation and ventricular tachycardia after administration of lidocaine or bretylium doses.

Onset and Duration   Onset: Immediate
Duration: 3 to 4 hours

Indications

- Seizures of eclampsia (toxemia of pregnancy)
- Torsades de pointes
- Bronchospasm from asthma

Contraindications

- Heart block

Adverse Reactions

- Diaphoresis
- Facial flushing
- Hypotension
- Depressed reflexes
- Hypothermia
- Reduced heart rate
- Circulatory collapse
- Respiratory depression

Drug Interactions   Central nervous system depressant effects may be enhanced if the patient is taking other CNS depressants.

Serious changes in cardiac function may occur with cardiac glycosides.

Dosage and Administration   **Seizure activity associated with pregnancy**

For severe pre-eclampsia or eclampsia, administer magnesium sulfate 2.0 g, IV/saline lock drip, diluted in 50 to 100 mL of normal saline (0.9), over 10 to 20 minutes. If seizures develop, continue, or recur in transport, repeat magnesium sulfate 2 g, IV/saline lock drip, diluted in 100 mL of normal saline (0.9), over 10 to 20 minutes.

Magnesium deficiency related to cardiac dysrhythmias, torsade's de pointe, or refractory ventricular fibrillation

2.0 g, IV/saline lock bolus, diluted in 10 mL of normal saline (0.9), over 2 minutes

Asthma   2.0 g, IV/saline lock drip, diluted in 50 to 100 mL of normal saline (0.9), over 10 to 20 minutes.

Special Considerations   Pregnancy safety: Magnesium sulfate is administered to treat toxemia of pregnancy. It is recommended that the drug not be administered in the 2 hours before delivery, if possible. IV calcium gluconate or calcium chloride should be available as an antagonist to magnesium if needed.

Convulsions may occur up to 48 hours after delivery, necessitating continued therapy. The "cure" for toxemia is delivery of the baby. Magnesium must be used with caution in patients with renal failure, since it is cleared by the kidneys and can reach toxic levels easily in those patients. Prophylactic administration of magnesium sulfate for patients with acute myocardial infarction should be considered.

Metaproterenol (Alupent)®

Class Sympathomimetic, bronchodilator

Description Metaproterenol relaxes the smooth muscles of the bronchial tree and peripheral vasculature by stimulating β_2-adrenergic receptors of the sympathetic nervous system. It activates adenyl cyclase, the enzyme that catalyzes the conversion of adenosine triphosphate to cyclic adenosine monophosphate.

Onset and Duration Onset: 5 minutes after inhalation
Duration: 4 to 6 hours

Indications

- Bronchial asthma
- Reversible bronchospasm (bronchitis, emphysema)

Contraindications

- Hypersensitivity
- Cardiac dysrhythmias
- Tachycardia caused by digitalis toxicity

Adverse Reactions

- Restlessness
- Tremor
- Palpitations
- Tachycardia
- Dysrhythmias
- Decreased blood pressure
- Coughing
- Facial flushing
- Diaphoresis

Drug Interactions Other sympathomimetics may exacerbate adverse cardiovascular effects. MAO inhibitors may potentiate hypotensive effects.
Beta blockers may antagonize metaproterenol.

Dosage and Administration **Adult**

Five percent (0.3 mL in 2.5-3.0 mL of normal saline [0.9]), nebulized, at a flow rate that will deliver the solution over 5 to 15 minutes. May be repeated twice (total of three doses).

Pediatric   Five percent (0.3 mL in 2.5-3.0 mL of normal saline [0.9]), by nebulizer, at a flow rate that will deliver the solution over 5 to 15 minutes.

Special Considerations   Pregnancy safety: Category C.

Monitor vital signs for hypotension and tachycardia.

Use with caution in patients with coronary artery disease and diabetes mellitus.

Methylprednisolone (Solu-Medrol)®

Class   Glucocorticoid

Description   Methylprednisolone is a synthetic steroid that suppresses acute and chronic inflammation and may alter the immune response. In addition, it potentiates vascular smooth muscle relaxation by beta-adrenergic agonists and may alter airway hyperactivity.

Onset and Duration   Onset: 1 to 2 hours

Duration: 8 to 24 hours

Indications

- Anaphylaxis
- Bronchodilator for unresponsive asthma
- Acute spinal cord injury
- Endocrine disorders
- Rheumatic disorders
- Dermatological diseases
- Allergic states

Contraindications

- Hypersensitivity
- Premature infants
- Systemic fungal infections
- Use with caution in patients with GI bleeding and diabetes mellitus

Adverse Reactions

- Headache
- Hypertension
- Sodium and water retention

- Hypokalemia
- Alkalosis
- Cataracts
- Psychosis
- Osteoporosis
- Peptic ulcer
- Impaired wound healing
- Development of cushingoid state

Drug Interactions   Hypoglycemic responses to insulin and oral hypoglycemic agents may be blunted.

Potassium-depleting agents may potentiate hypokalemia induced by corticosteroids.

Dosage and Administration   125 mg, IV/saline lock bolus, slowly, over 2 minutes, or IM

Special Considerations   Pregnancy safety: Not established.

May mask some signs of infection

Oxygen (O_2)
Class   Gas
Actions   Necessary for cellular metabolism.
Indications   Hypoxia.
Contraindications   None.
Precautions   Use cautiously in patients with COPD, humidify when providing high-flow rates.
Side Effects   Drying of mucous membranes.
Dosage   Cardiac arrest: 100%; other critical patients: 100%; COPD: 35%.
Pediatric Dosage   24 to 100% as required.
Routes   Inhalation.

Racemic Epinephrine (Micronefrin) (Vaponefrin)®
Class   Sympathomimetic
Actions   Bronchodilation, increases heart rate, increases cardiac contractile force.
Indications   Croup (laryngotracheobronchitis).
Contraindications   Epiglottitis, hypersensitivity to the drug.
Precautions   Vital signs should be constantly monitored. Should be used only once in the prehospital setting.
Side Effects   Palpitations, anxiety, headache.

Dosage   0.5 to 0.75 mL of a 2.25% solution in 2.0 mL normal saline.

Pediatric Dosage   0.25 to 0.75 mL of a 2.25% solution in 2.0 mL normal saline.

Routes   Inhalation only (small-volume nebulizer).

Terbutaline (Brethine)

Class   Sympathomimetic

Actions   Bronchodilator-increases heart rate.

Indications   Bronchial asthma, reversible bronchospasm associated with COPD, preterm labor.

Contraindications   Patients with known hypersensitivity to the drug.

Precautions   Blood pressure, pulse, and ECG must be constantly monitored.

Side Effects   Palpitations, tachycardia, and PVCs, anxiety, tremor, and headache.

Dosage   Metered-dose inhaler: two inhalations, 1 minute apart.

   Subcutaneous injection: 0.25 mg; may be repeated in 15 to 30 minutes.

   Preterm labor: 0.25 mg IM or IV. May be repeated in 15 to 30 minutes as needed

Pediatric Dosage   0.01 mg/kg subcutaneously.

Routes   Inhalation, subcutaneous injection, IV (preterm labor only).

REVIEW QUESTIONS

1. The regions of the body associated with the parasympathetic nervous system are:
   A. thoracolumbar region.
   B. the cranial and sacral regions of the spinal cord.
   C. cervical spinal region.
   D. the brain.

Correct answer is b.

2. The regions of the body associated with the sympathetic nervous system are:
   A. thoracolumbar region.
   B. the cranial and sacral regions of the spinal cord.
   C. cervical spinal region.
   D. the brain.

Correct answer is a.

3. The _____ is a form of respiratory drive in which the body uses oxygen chemoreceptors instead of carbon dioxide receptors to regulate the respiratory cycle.

A. apneustic drive

B. hypoxic drive

C. chemoreceptor drive

D. chemotaxic drive

Correct answer is b.

4. These drugs help expel bronchial secretions from the respiratory tract by decreasing their viscosity, thus facilitating removal, and by increasing the amount of respiratory tract fluid, thus exerting a demulcent action on the mucosal lining. Most expectorants increase secretions through reflex irritation of the bronchial mucosa.

A. Decongestant.

B. Bronchodilator.

C. Expectorant.

D. Mucolytic.

Correct answer is c.

5. _____ is a sympathomimetic that is selective for β_2-adrenergic receptors. It relaxes smooth muscles of the bronchial tree and peripheral vasculature by stimulating adrenergic receptors of the sympathetic nervous system.

A. Albuterol sulfate

B. Methylprednisone

C. Magnesium sulfate

D. Furosemide

Correct answer is a.

6. The medication known as a xanthine dilator:

A. Albuterol sulfate

B. Methylprednisone

C. Magnesium sulfate

D. Theophylline

Correct answer is d.

7. Racemic epinephrine is a medication class known as:

   A. bronchodilator.
   B. steroid.
   C. glucocorticoid.
   D. xanthine.

Correct answer is a.

8. _____ prevents the physiological actions of histamine by preventing histamine from reaching H_1- and H_2-receptor sites.

   A. Diphenhydramine
   B. Epinephrine
   C. Racemic epinephrine
   D. Magnesium sulfate

Correct answer is a.

9. Asthma, reversible bronchospasm associated with chronic bronchitis, and emphysema are treated with which medication in an emergency setting?

   A. Albuterol sulfate
   B. Ipratropium bromide
   C. Isoetharine
   D. All of the above

Correct answer is d.

10. Contraindications for epinephrine include:

    A. hypersensitivity
    B. hypovolemic shock
    C. narrow angle glaucoma
    D. All of the above

Correct answer is d.

11. The primary neurochemical mediator of both sympathetic and parasympathetic preganglionic neurons is:

    A. acetylcholine.
    B. norepinephrine.
    C. Both a and b are correct.
    D. None of the above.

Correct answer is a.

12. _____ is a neurochemical mediator in the central nervous system and probably also in some neurons in the superior cervical ganglion and the kidney.

   A. Norepinephrine
   B. Acetylcholine
   C. Dopamine
   D. Epinephrine

Correct answer is c.

13. Norepinephrine, epinephrine, and dopamine are sometimes collectively referred to as catecholamines.

   A. True
   B. False

Correct answer is a.

14. A relatively β_2 selective adrenergic bronchodilator:

   A. Albuterol sulfate
   B. Dexamethasone
   C. Aminophylline
   D. Hexadrol

Correct answer is a.

15. The correct dose for metaproterenol for an adult experiencing an asthma attack is:

   A. 3.0 mL of 5% metaproterenol inhalation solution diluted in 2.5 mL normal saline.
   B. 0.3 mL of 5% metaproterenol inhalation solution diluted in 2.5 mL normal saline.
   C. 1.5 mL of 5% metaproterenol inhalation solution diluted in 2.5 mL normal saline.
   D. 0.003 mL of 5% metaproterenol inhalation solution diluted in 2.5 mL normal saline.

Correct answer is b.

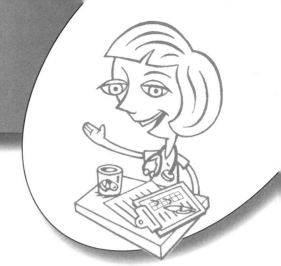

chapter 7

Respiratory Emergencies

LEARNING OBJECTIVES

At the end of this chapter, you will be able to:

1. Describe the components of a respiratory assessment.

2. Recognize clinical manifestations associated with common respiratory disorders.

3. List medical interventions for common respiratory disorders.

4. Evaluate interventions carried out for common respiratory disorders.

KEY TERMS

Apnea	Hyperpnea
Apneustic breathing	Hyperventilation
Acute respiratory distress syndrome	Kussmaul's respirations
Ataxic respirations	Narcotic overdose
Biot's respirations	Orthopnea
Bradypnea	Pleural friction rub
Central neurogenic hyperventilation	Pulmonary embolism
Cheyne-Stokes respirations	Re-expansion pulmonary edema
Crackles	Rhonchi
Dyspnea	Tachypnea
Eupnea	Wheezing
High altitude pulmonary edema	

Scenario

You and your partner have responded to an adult male having difficulty breathing. Upon arrival you find a 56-year-old male patient with a history of asthma who has been wheezing all day and has not responded to home nebulizer treatments. He has had a "cold" with cough and low-grade fever for several days. BP is 104/60, pulse 110, and respiration rate is 24 breaths per minute with audible wheezing. He has wheezing bilaterally. Pulse oximeter reading is 92%. You are 30 minutes from the hospital.

What would your treatment be?

Respiratory Patterns

TABLE 7-1 Respiratory Patterns

Pattern	Description
Eupnea	Normal rate and depth
Tachypnea	Used to describe rapid rate regardless of depth. (Depth is variable.)
Hyperventilation	Used to describe increased depth regardless of rate. (Rate is variable.) Depth exceeds metabolic demands of the body, so patient may have high oxygen (O_2) and low carbon dioxide content.

TABLE 7-1 Respiratory Patterns (continued)	
Pattern	**Description**
Hyperpnea	Both rate and depth are increased but they meet the metabolic demands of the body, therefore O_2 and carbon dioxide levels may be normal.
Kussmaul's respirations	Rapid and deep breathing without pauses. Patient appears to be air hungry, gasping to breath. Usually associated with states of acidosis.
Dyspnea	Subjective sensation of difficult or labored breathing.
Orthopnea	Sensation of dyspnea when lying down.
Bradypnea	Used to describe decreased rate regardless of depth. (Depth is variable.)
Apnea	Absence of breathing.
Biot's respirations	Fast and deep breathing punctuated by periods of apnea. Related to damage to the medulla oblongata from strokes or trauma. May also be seen in meningitis.
Ataxic respirations	Irregular, random pattern of deep and shallow respirations with irregular apneic periods. Usually a poor indicator of prognosis associated with increased intracranial pressure.
Central neurogenic hyperventilation	Very deep and rapid respirations with no apneic periods associated with increased intracranial pressure.
Apneustic breathing	Prolonged inspiratory and/or expiratory pause of 2-3 seconds. This usually signifies the presence of brainstem lesions usually at the level of the pons.
Cheyne-Stoke respirations	Rhythmic crescendo and decrescendo of rate and depth of respiration, which includes brief periods of apnea. Usually associated with increases of carbon dioxide in the cerebrum.

Lung Sounds

TABLE 7-2 Lung Sounds		
Breath Sound	**Description**	**Significance**
Wheezing	A whistling or musical sound	Caused by narrowing of the lower or smaller airways.
Rhonchi	A snoring, low-pitched sound	Caused by narrowing of the larger upper airways.
Crackles	Small popping sounds	Produced by the movement of air through secretions or lightly closed airways.
Pleural friction rub	Grating sound which may be compared to rubbing your hair between your fingers near your ear that is heard with inspiration and expiration.	Caused by inflammation of the pleural surfaces. The inflamed surfaces rub together during the respiratory cycle to produce this sound.

Asthma

Asthma is a reversible bronchiolar airway constriction often associated with allergies, but not always. In some people, asthma attacks can be triggered by exertion or excitement as well. In asthma, bronchiolar smooth muscle contracts uncontrollably producing "wheezing." In allergic individuals, the bronchiolar constriction is the result of histamine release in the lungs in response to an allergen.

Because bronchioles constrict, asthma causes difficulty with exhalation. Recall that during inspiration, the elastic lung airways are literally "pulled" open as the lungs expand allowing air to enter relatively unobstructed. However, in response to histamine release, the airways swell and secrete thick mucus. These events, when combined with smooth muscle contraction, cause the airways to close completely during exhalation making it difficult to expire the inhaled air. This "trapped air" remains in the lungs raising the functional residual capacity (FRV) and making it more difficult to inhale sufficient air with the next breath. As trapped air volume increases, the inspiratory reserve decreases accordingly making it difficult to "turn over" enough of the FRV to maintain blood oxygenation and carbon dioxide removal. In extreme cases, suffocation can result. Since the bronchiolar constriction is reversible, treatment with a bronchodilator (epinephrine in extreme cases) gives relief or the constriction may subside on its own in time.

Chronic Obstructive Pulmonary Disease

TABLE 7-3 Chronic Obstructive Pulmonary Disease Comparison	
Chronic Bronchitis	**Emphysema**
"Blue bloater"	"Pink puffer"
Productive cough	Cough uncommon
Stocky build	Thin
Onset 40-50 years	Onset 50-75 years
Normal respiratory rate	Tachypnea
Hypoxemia	PaO_2 normal or slightly
Increased PaO_2	$PaCO_2$ low or normal until the end
Cyanosis	Barrel chest
Polycythemia	Accessory muscle use

TABLE 7-3 Chronic Obstructive Pulmonary Disease Comparison (continued)	
Chronic Bronchitis	**Emphysema**
Cor Pulmonale	Leans forward while sitting
Peripheral edema	Pursed-lip breathing
Risk for pulmonary embolism	Hyperesonance on percussion
Enlarged heart on x-ray	Lung over-inflation and low diaphragm on x-ray

Chronic Bronchitis

Somewhat like asthma, in chronic bronchitis the conducting airways are inflamed chronically by an irritant and swell with heavy mucus secretion. These inflamed airways close during exhalation causing air trapping. In many cases the air trapping is sufficient to cause a "barrel-chested" appearance over the course of the disease (Figure 7-1).

Because of poor lung ventilation, patients are often hypoxic and exhibit cyanosis and hypercapnia. The hypercapnia is particularly serious since it develops over a long time and the respiratory centers of the brain adapt to the high carbon dioxide (CO_2) levels to the extent that these patients depend upon their "back up" system to trigger breathing. This back-up system relies on low oxygen (O_2) to stimulate breathing. (This is known as hypoxic drive.) The hyper-inflated lungs of these patients increases resistance to blood flow through the pulmonary capillaries on the surfaces of the distended alveoli. This can lead to pulmonary artery hypertension (PAH) and eventually to cor pulmonale (right CHF).

Emphysema

It is important to note that "pure" emphysema is rarely encountered. It usually occurs in conjunction with bronchitis with irritant particles being the cause of both.

Should emphysema occur singularly, it results in a loss of respiratory surface instead of airway obstruction. In fact, an emphysemics lung volume may stay the same or increase but the loss of respiratory membrane surface impairs gas exchange. These individuals may even show diminished breath sounds as airways are lost or fused together. Since capillaries occur on alveolar surfaces, they too may be lost as the disease progresses. This can also increase resistance causing PAH and right CHF.

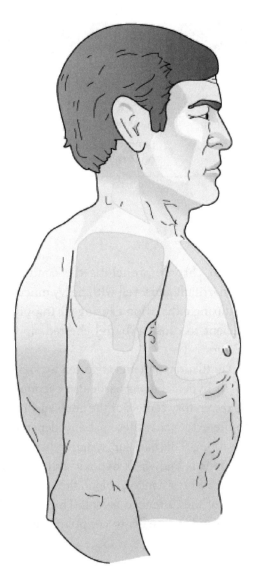

FIGURE 7-1 • "Barrel-chested" appearance.
Reproduced with permission from DeTurk WE, Cahalin LP, eds. *Cardiovascular and Pulmonary Physical Therapy: An Evidence-Based Approach.* 2011. New York: Copyright © McGraw-Hill Education. All rights reserved.

Since respiratory surface is lost, compensation of gas exchange is possible. Emphysemics frequently use "pursed lip breathing" as compensation. By exhaling against pursed lips, airway pressures are increased above normal and this helps prevent their collapse during exhalation. It also raises the air pressure in remaining alveoli literally driving more O_2 into blood.

Pulmonary Edema

I. Cardiogenic Pulmonary Edema

Pathophysiology

This is caused by rapid transudation of fluid into lungs secondary to increased pulmonary wedge pressure, without time for compensation of the pulmonary bed. Increased wedge pressure translates to increased pulmonary venous pressure and elevated microvascular pressure, leading to transudation of fluid (Starling's forces at work!). This can occur at wedge pressures as low as 18 mm Hg or not until > 25 mm Hg if chronic condition has resulted in increased lymphatic drainage capacity.

Etiology

A. Heart muscle

1. Systolic dysfunction is the most common cause of pulmonary edema. This can be due to coronary artery disease (CAD), hypertension (HTN), valvular disease, idiopathic dilated cardiomyopathy, toxins, hypothyroidism, and viral myocarditis. If condition is somewhat chronic, volume overload is exacerbated by renin angiotensin system upregulation due to decreased forward flow.

2. Diastolic dysfunction is the increase in ventricular stiffness which impairs filling, leading to proximal pressure rise. Causes include hypertrophic and restrictive cardiomyopathies, ischemia, and hypertensive crises.

B. Valvular problems

1. Mitral stenosis usually due to rheumatic heart disease.

2. Aortic stenosis which causes pulmonary edema by requiring elevated left ventricular end-diastolic (LVED) pressure filling. This translates to high pulmonary pressures and cardiac ischemia due to impaired diastolic coronary artery filling.

3. Aortic regurgitation acutely can be seen in infective endocarditis or aortic dissection.

C. Other causes

1. Renal artery stenosis: In some cases, pulmonary edema has been the presenting sign of renal artery stenosis.

2. Atrial myxoma (connective tissue tumor), intra-cardiac thrombus impeding left atrial outflow track, congenital membrane in left atrium (cor triatriatum).

Diagnosis

1. History and physical examination of the patient.
2. ECG: Ischemic changes are consistent with CAD. Can also see depressed T waves, global T-wave inversions, and marked QT interval prolongation unrelated to ischemia that resolve within 1 to 7 days.
3. Echocardiogram (in-hospital).

Treatment

1. Supplemental oxygen
2. CPAP
3. Diuretics: Lasix or other loop diuretics. Dosage should be at least 40 mg IV but often higher are doses needed, especially if patient is already on diuretics at home. Peak diuresis is in 30 minutes. Furosemide initially causes vasodilation prior to onset of diuresis. Chronic CHF can occasionally see transient arteriolar vasoconstriction and increased BP due to increase in plasma renin and norepinephrine levels.

What Went Wrong? IV loop diuretics, especially furosemide, have been used for many years as the cornerstone of treatment in patients who present with cardiogenic pulmonary edema. These medications produce a decrease in preload by inhibiting sodium chloride reabsorption in the ascending loop of Henle, which promotes increases in urine volume and excretion; however, because patients who develop cardiogenic pulmonary edema have elevated systemic vascular resistance (afterload), renal perfusion is markedly diminished. As a result, diuretics have a significantly delayed effect, often taking 45 to 120 minutes to produce effective diuresis. Further complicating the use of diuretics in these patients is evidence that as many as 40% of patients who present with cardiogenic pulmonary edema have intravascular euvolemia or hypovolemia. The use of diuretics in these patients may be associated with adverse effects, including electrolyte abnormalities and hypotension by over diuresis.

4. Morphine: Dosage is usually 2 to 5 mg over 3 minutes that can be repeated in 15 minutes if necessary. Morphine decreases patient anxiety and work of breathing, thereby limiting sympathetic outflow and aiding in arteriolar and venous dilatation.
5. Vasodilators: Nitroglycerin or nitroprusside is especially helpful for HTN emergency, acute aortic or mitral regurgitation, and acute ventricular septal wall defect.

6. Position: Sit patient upright.
7. Positive pressure ventilation: This decreases venous return and increases pressure gradient between LV and extrathoracic arteries. To be used with caution as one study showed increased incidence of deterioration requiring intubation when compared with high dose nitrate group.

II. Noncardiogenic pulmonary edema

Noncardiogenic pulmonary edema is defined as radiographic evidence of alveolar fluid accumulation without elevated pulmonary capillary-wedge pressure.*

Pathophysiology

Alveolar-capillary membrane becomes damaged and leaky, resulting in movement of proteins and water into the interstitial space.

Etiologies

1. Acute respiratory distress syndrome (ARDS): There are multiple etiologies including sepsis, DIC, inhaled toxins, radiation pneumonia, inhalation of high oxygen concentrations, and severe trauma (thoracic or otherwise). ARDS often occurs within the first 2 hours of an inciting event, but can occur as late as 1 to 3 days later. X-rays typically show a bilateral alveolar filling pattern. In-hospital treatment includes treating the underlying cause. High frequency, low volume ventilation with diuresis is proven to be beneficial.

2. Re-expansion pulmonary edema: This can occur after re-expansion of pneumothorax or following removal of large amounts of pleural fluid (> 1.0-1.5 L). This can be seen within an hour in 64% of the patients. Ongoing for 24 to 48 hrs but symptoms can last up to 5 days. Pathophysiology is unknown but worse in patients with chronic collapse. Supportive treatment is applied. Mortality has been reported as high as 20%.

3. High-altitude pulmonary edema: Etiology is unclear but it is thought to be due to unequal pulmonary vasoconstriction and over-perfusion of remaining vessels. Support patient and move to lower altitudes.

4. Narcotic overdose: Overdose of opiates such as, heroin or methadone. Usually occurs within 2 hours of injection. Pathophysiology is unknown

---

*Hypoalbuminemia does not cause pulmonary edema.

but is believed to be due to direct toxicity, hypoxia, hyperventilation, or cerebral edema. Supportive measures for patient are indicated.

5. Pulmonary embolism: Treatment aimed at anticoagulation and supportive measures.

What Went Wrong?   Pulmonary edema can be confused with diffuse alveolar hemorrhage or lymphangitic spread of cancer. Not all cases of diffuse alveolar hemorrhage present with hemoptysis, but clues to diagnosis may be in unexplained hematocrit drop. Lymphangitic spread of tumors most often seen with lymphoma or acute leukemia, but solid tumors can behave this way.

Diagnosis

1. History and physical examination.
2. ABG can be helpful.

III. Neurogenic

Presentation

Hypoxia, tachypnea, diffuse rales, frothy sputum or hemoptysis in setting of neurologic disorders or procedures. Occurs within minutes to hours of severe CNS insult and can be confused with aspiration pneumonitis/pneumonia.

Common CNS injuries

Epileptic seizures, head injury, cerebral hemorrhage (subarachnoid or intracerebral). In head injuries, pulmonary edema is seen with elevated intracranial pressures.

Pathophysiology

This is likely due to sympathetic activation causing pulmonary vasoconstriction and increased vascular permeability.

Pneumonia

Common Causes

It consists of an alveolar inflammation caused by infectious or noninfectious pathogens. Its classification is based on the contaminant source.

Community Acquired

Refers to pneumonia contracted outside the hospital environment. Most common pathogens associated with community acquired pneumonia include

Streptococcus pneumoniae, Haemophilus influenzae, Mycoplasma pneumoniae. It spreads by fluid and contact transmission.

Hospital Acquired

Leading cause of nosocomial pneumonia is aspiration pneumonia.

1. Leads to acute mechanical airway constriction.
2. Cellular debris in air spaces between large airways and alveoli.
3. Evidence of an inflammatory response.
4. Evidence of pulmonary microvasculature and lung parenchyma.

Types of Aspiration Pneumonia

1. Chemical aspiration reaches the pleura in about 18 seconds, Type I alveolar cells die first, then type II alveolar cells. Causes include:
   - Hydrochloric acid with a pH < 2.5
   - Bile
   - Mineral oil
   - Gasoline
2. Inert fluid aspiration pH > 3.0. Causes include:
   - Fresh water
   - Saltwater
   - Nasogastric feedings
3. Particulate aspiration may result in obstructive atelectasis. Chest x-ray may show mediastinal shift. Bronchoscopy is usually needed to remove the material. Causes include:
   - Peanuts, teeth, or food
4. Bacterial aspiration causes include:
   - Poor dental hygiene resulting in mixed anaerobe bacterial pneumonia.

Ventilator-Associated Pneumonia

Ventilator-associated pneumonia (VAPS) occurs within 48 to 72 hours of endotracheal intubation. It results from antibiotic-resistant pathogens, such as:

1. *Staphylococcus aureus*
2. *Pseudomonas aeruginosa*

3. *Acinetobacter* species

4. *Enterobacter* species

Pathophysiology

Pneumonia is a restrictive lung disease that is characterized by inflammation of lung parenchyma with exudative solidification or consolidation and results in:

- Decreased lung compliance
- Abnormal gas exchange
- Ventilation–perfusion (V/Q) mismatch
- Shunt

Permanent parenchymal lung damage results from infection with some organisms depending on the degree of necrotizing action they have.

- Gram-negative bacteria have a greater tendency for necrotizing action.
- Gram-positive bacteria have a lesser tendency than the gram-negative bacteria.

The difference between bacterial and viral pneumonia is as follows:

1. Bacterial pneumonia
   - There is complete alveolar consolidation.
   - Impaired mucociliary clearance.
2. Viral pneumonia
   - Affects the airways more than the alveolar spaces.

Potential Complications

1. Lung abscess
2. Bronchiectasis
3. Empyema
4. Pericarditis and/or endocarditis
5. ARDS
6. Formation of cysts and bullae
7. Pneumothorax
8. Pleural effusion
9. Respiratory failure
10. Reye's syndrome
11. Pulmonary fibrosis

12. Blood sepsis

13. Septic shock

In-hospital Diagnosis

- Laboratory: Only 30% to 60% of pneumonia patients have the pathogenic organism identified.
- Complete blood chemistry
  - leukocytosis
    - initially prevalent in bacterial pneumonia
    - in nonbacterial pneumonia, the WBC is normal.
- Blood cultures
  - used to establish the etiology of the infection.
- Serologic tests-mostly indicate a viral pneumonia.
  - influenza
  - para influenza
  - RSV
  - cytomegalovirus
  - Pneumonitis
- Sputum culture collected before the use of antibiotics.
  - Gram stain: identifies the general category of the involved bacteria.
  - culture: identifies the specific pathogen.
  - sensitivity: identifies the antibiotic that the bacteria are susceptible to.
- Chest x-ray
  - increased density
  - air bronchograms
  - bacterial pneumonia: lobar pneumonia
  - viral pneumonia: unilateral or bilateral interstitial infiltrates.
  - gastric pneumonia: bilateral patchy airspace consolidation favoring perihilar or basal regions.
  - necrotizing pneumonia: areas of radiolucency caused by lung destruction.
  - syphilis: white-out pneumonia.

Physical Examination
Acute Bacterial Pneumonia

- Sudden onset of symptoms
  - chills
  - high fever
  - hacking cough
- Producing purulent and abundant pink, brown, or yellow sputum.
  - headaches
  - skin rashes
  - nausea
  - diarrhea
- Patients with a chronic pulmonary disease or multiple lung fields are affected.
  - chest pain, usually pleuritic
  - dyspnea
- Other signs
  - unilateral chest expansion
  - tactile fremitus
  - dullness to percussion
- Auscultation
  - decreased breath sounds
  - rales or wheezes
  - coarse crackles
  - a pleuritic friction rub
  - cyanosis
  - accessory muscle
  - increase heart rate
  - increase respiratory rate

Viral or Mycoplasma Pneumoniae

- Gradual onset of symptoms
  - low-grade fever
  - scant, mucoid sputum

- chills
- chest pain
- lobar or segmental consolidation

Treatment

1. Oxygen, if needed
2. Continuous positive airflow pressure (CPAP), as per local protocol
3. Pain medications as needed for chest pain
4. Aerosol therapy if indicated
5. Chest physical therapy
6. IV fluids, treatment of dehydration

Respiratory Failure

Respiratory failure is a syndrome in which the respiratory system fails in one or both of its gas exchange functions: oxygenation and carbon dioxide elimination. In medicine, respiratory failure is defined as a PaO_2 value of less than 60 mm Hg while breathing air or a $PaCO_2$ of more than 50 mm Hg. Furthermore, respiratory failure may be acute or chronic. While acute respiratory failure is characterized by life-threatening derangements in arterial blood gases (ABG) and acid–base status, the manifestations of chronic respiratory failure are less dramatic and may not be as readily apparent.

Classification of Respiratory Failure

Respiratory failure may be classified as hypoxemic or hypercapnic and may be either acute or chronic.

Hypoxemic respiratory failure (type I) is characterized by a PaO_2 of less than 60 mm Hg with a normal or low $PaCO_2$. This is the most common form of respiratory failure, and it can be associated with virtually all acute diseases of the lung, which generally involve fluid filling or collapse of alveolar units. Some examples of type I respiratory failure is cardiogenic or noncardiogenic pulmonary edema, pneumonia, and pulmonary hemorrhage.

Hypercapnic respiratory failure (type II) is characterized by a $PaCO_2$ of more than 50 mm Hg. Hypoxemia is common in patients with hypercapnic respiratory failure who are breathing room air. The pH depends on the level of bicarbonate, which, in turn, is dependent on the duration of hypercapnia. Common etiologies include drug overdose, neuromuscular disease, chest wall abnormalities, and severe airway disorders (ie, asthma, COPD).

Distinctions Between Acute and Chronic Respiratory Failure

Acute hypercapnic respiratory failure develops over minutes to hours; therefore, pH is less than 7.3. Chronic respiratory failure develops over several days or longer, allowing time for renal compensation and an increase in bicarbonate concentration. Therefore, the pH usually is only slightly decreased.

The distinction between acute and chronic hypoxemic respiratory failure cannot readily be made on the basis of ABGs. The clinical markers of chronic hypoxemia, such as polycythemia or cor pulmonale, suggest a long-standing disorder.

Pathophysiology

Respiratory failure can arise from an abnormality in any of the components of the respiratory system, including the airways, alveoli, CNS, peripheral nervous system, respiratory muscles, and chest wall. Patients who have hypoperfusion secondary to cardiogenic, hypovolemic, or septic shock often present with respiratory failure.

Hypoxemic respiratory failure: The pathophysiologic mechanisms that account for the hypoxemia observed in a wide variety of diseases are V/Q mismatch and shunt. These two mechanisms lead to widening of the alveolar-arterial oxygen difference, which normally is less than 15 mm Hg. With V/Q mismatch, the areas of low ventilation relative to perfusion (low V/Q units) contribute to hypoxemia. An intrapulmonary or intracardiac shunt causes mixed venous (deoxygenated) blood to bypass ventilated alveoli and results in venous admixture. The distinction between V/Q mismatch and shunt can be made by assessing the response to oxygen supplementation or calculating the shunt fraction following inhalation of 100% oxygen. In most patients with hypoxemic respiratory failure, these two mechanisms coexist.

Hypercapnic respiratory failure: A decrease in alveolar ventilation can result from a reduction in overall (minute) ventilation or an increase in the proportion of dead space ventilation. A reduction in minute ventilation is observed primarily in the setting of neuromuscular disorders and CNS depression. In pure hypercapnic respiratory failure, the hypoxemia is easily corrected with O_2 therapy.

The diagnosis of acute or chronic respiratory failure begins with clinical suspicion of its presence. Confirmation of the diagnosis is based on ABG analysis.

Evaluation of an underlying cause must be initiated early, frequently in the presence of concurrent treatment for acute respiratory failure.

- The cause of respiratory failure often is evident after a careful history and physical examination.

- Cardiogenic pulmonary edema usually develops in the context of a history of left ventricular dysfunction or valvular heart disease.

- A history of previous cardiac disease, recent symptoms of chest pain, paroxysmal nocturnal dyspnea, and orthopnea suggest cardiogenic pulmonary edema.

- Noncardiogenic edema (ie, acute respiratory distress syndrome [ARDS]) occurs in typical clinical contexts such as sepsis, trauma, aspiration, pneumonia, pancreatitis, drug toxicity, and multiple transfusions.

Physical Examination

The signs and symptoms of acute respiratory failure reflect the underlying disease process and the associated hypoxemia or hypercapnia. Localized pulmonary findings reflecting the acute cause of hypoxemia, such as pneumonia, pulmonary edema, asthma, or COPD, may be readily apparent. In patients with ARDS, the manifestations may be remote from the thorax, such as abdominal pain or long-bone fracture. Neurological manifestations include restlessness, anxiety, confusion, seizures, or coma.

- Asterixis may be observed with severe hypercapnia. Tachycardia and a variety of arrhythmias may result from hypoxemia and acidosis.

- Once respiratory failure is suspected on clinical grounds, ABG analysis should be performed to confirm the diagnosis and to assist in the distinction between acute and chronic forms. This helps assess the severity of respiratory failure and also helps guide management.

- Cyanosis, a bluish color of skin and mucous membranes, indicates hypoxemia. Visible cyanosis typically is present when the concentration of deoxygenated hemoglobin in the capillaries or tissues is at least 5 g/dL.

- Dyspnea, an uncomfortable sensation of breathing, often accompanies respiratory failure. Excessive respiratory effort, vagal receptors, and chemical stimuli (hypoxemia and/or hypercapnia) all may contribute to the sensation of dyspnea.

- Both confusion and somnolence may occur in respiratory failure. Myoclonus and seizures may occur with severe hypoxemia. Polycythemia is a complication of long-standing hypoxemia.

- Pulmonary hypertension frequently is present in chronic respiratory failure. Alveolar hypoxemia potentiated by hypercapnia causes pulmonary arteriolar constriction. If chronic, this is accompanied by hypertrophy and hyperplasia of the affected smooth muscles and narrowing of the pulmonary arterial bed. The increased pulmonary vascular resistance increases afterload of the right ventricle, which may induce right ventricular failure. This, in turn, causes enlargement of the liver and peripheral edema. The entire sequence is known as cor pulmonale.
- Criteria for the diagnosis of ARDS
  - clinical presentation: Tachypnea and dyspnea; crackles upon auscultation
  - clinical setting: Direct insult (aspiration) or systemic process causing lung injury (sepsis)
  - radiologic appearance: Three-quadrant or 4-quadrant alveolar flooding
  - lung mechanics: Diminished compliance (< 40 mL/cm water)
  - gas exchange: Severe hypoxia refractory to O_2 therapy (PaO_2/FIO_2 < 200)
  - normal pulmonary vascular properties: Pulmonary capillary wedge pressure < 18 mm Hg

Causes

These diseases can be grouped according to the primary abnormality and the individual components of the respiratory system, as follows:

- Central nervous system disorders
  - a variety of pharmacological, structural, and metabolic disorders of the CNS are characterized by depression of the neural drive to breathe.
  - this may lead to acute or chronic hypoventilation and hypercapnia.
  - examples include tumors or vascular abnormalities involving the brain stem, an overdose of narcotic or sedative and metabolic disorders such as myxedema or chronic metabolic alkalosis.
- Disorders of the peripheral nervous system, respiratory muscles, and chest wall
  - these disorders lead to an inability to maintain a level of minute ventilation appropriate for the rate of carbon dioxide production.
  - concomitant hypoxemia and hypercapnia occur.
  - examples include Guillain-Barré syndrome, muscular dystrophy, myasthenia gravis, severe kyphoscoliosis, and morbid obesity.

- Abnormalities of the airways
  - severe airway obstruction is a common cause of acute and chronic hypercapnia.
  - examples of upper airway disorders are acute epiglottitis and tumors involving the trachea; lower airway disorders include COPD, asthma, and cystic fibrosis.
- Abnormalities of the alveoli
  - the diseases are characterized by diffuse alveolar filling, frequently resulting in hypoxemic respiratory failure, although hypercapnia may complicate the clinical picture.
  - common examples are cardiogenic and noncardiogenic pulmonary edema, aspiration pneumonia, or extensive pulmonary hemorrhage. These disorders are associated with intrapulmonary shunt and an increased work of breathing.
- Common causes of type I (hypoxemic) respiratory failure
  - chronic bronchitis and emphysema (COPD)
  - pneumonia
  - pulmonary edema
  - pulmonary fibrosis
  - asthma
  - pneumothorax
  - pulmonary embolism
  - pulmonary arterial hypertension
  - pneumoconiosis
  - granulomatous lung diseases
  - cyanotic congenital heart disease
  - bronchiectasis
  - ARDS
  - fat embolism syndrome
  - kyphoscoliosis
  - obesity
- Common causes of type II (hypercapnic) respiratory failure
  - chronic bronchitis and emphysema (COPD)
  - severe asthma

- drug overdose
- poisonings
- myasthenia gravis
- polyneuropathy
- poliomyelitis
- primary muscle disorders
- porphyria
- cervical cordotomy
- head and cervical cord injury
- primary alveolar hypoventilation
- obesity hypoventilation syndrome
- pulmonary edema
- ARDS
- myxedema
- tetanus

Treatment

Hypoxemia is the major immediate threat to organ function. Therefore, the first objective in the management of respiratory failure is to reverse and/or prevent tissue hypoxia. Hypercapnia unaccompanied by hypoxemia generally is well tolerated and probably is not a threat to organ function unless accompanied by severe acidosis. Many experts believe that hypercapnia should be tolerated until the arterial blood pH falls below 7.2. Appropriate management of the underlying disease obviously is an important component in the management of respiratory failure.

A patient with acute respiratory failure generally should be admitted to a respiratory care or intensive care unit. Most patients with chronic respiratory failure are treated at home with oxygen supplementation and/or ventilatory assist devices along with therapy for their underlying disease.

- Airway management
  - assurance of an adequate airway is vital in a patient with acute respiratory distress.
  - the most common indication for endotracheal intubation (ETT) is respiratory failure.

- ETT serves as an interface between the patient and the ventilator.
  - another indication for ETT is airway protection in patients with altered mental status.
- Correction of hypoxemia
  - after securing an airway, attention must turn to correcting the underlying hypoxemia, the most life-threatening facet of acute respiratory failure.
  - the goal is to assure adequate O_2 delivery to tissues, generally achieved with a PaO_2 of 60 mm Hg or arterial oxygen saturation (SaO_2) of greater than 90%.
  - Supplemental oxygen is administered via nasal prongs or face mask; however, in patients with severe hypoxemia, intubation and mechanical ventilation often are required.
- Coexistent hypercapnia and respiratory acidosis may need to be addressed. This is done by correcting the underlying cause or providing ventilatory assistance.
  - mechanical ventilation is used for two essential reasons:
    - to increase PaO_2 and
    - to lower $PaCO_2$. Mechanical ventilation also rests the respiratory muscles and is an appropriate therapy for respiratory muscle fatigue.
- After the patient's hypoxemia is corrected, and the ventilatory and hemodynamic status have stabilized, every attempt should be made to identify and correct the underlying pathophysiologic process that led to respiratory failure in the first place.
- The specific treatment depends on the etiology of respiratory failure.

REVIEW QUESTIONS

1. **The most reliable indicator of hypoxemia in the respiratory patient is**
   A. the level of consciousness.
   B. the end-tidal volume.
   C. the inspiratory breath sounds.
   D. the presence/absence of wheezing.

Correct answer is a.

2. The chronic overproduction of bronchial secretions with a productive cough is indicative of emphysema.

   A. True.
   B. False.

Correct answer is b.

3. Emphysema:

   A. is the chronic destruction of alveolar walls resulting in the build-up of carbon dioxide levels.
   B. is often seem after long-term bronchitis.
   C. a and b are correct.
   D. None of the above.

Correct answer is a.

4. The constriction of smooth bronchial muscles and a build-up of mucous plugs is most closely associated with:

   A. chronic bronchitis.
   B. emphysema.
   C. cardiogenic shock.
   D. asthma.

Correct answer is a.

5. If a patient with a COPD history is experiencing difficulty breathing and becoming hypoxic, the paramedic should:

   A. treat with low concentration O_2 via nasal cannula.
   B. treat with high concentration O_2 via nonrebreather mask.
   C. withhold all O_2 hypoxic drive will kick in any second.
   D. treat with medium concentration O_2 via a venturi mask.

Correct answer is b.

6. The asthma patient should be treated according to cause and location. In general, however, all asthma patients should receive humidified oxygen, IV hydration if prolonged, and psychological support.

   A. True.
   B. False.

Correct answer is a.

7. Respiratory disorders are extremely common. They are divided into two categories: acute and chronic.

   A. True.
   B. False.

Correct answer is a.

8. The disease process that affects patients over 40 years of age, with a long-term history of cigarette smoking, and a history of recurrent respiratory tract infections, is most likely:

   A. emphysema.
   B. asthma.
   C. cardiomyopathy.
   D. bronchitis.

Correct answer is a.

9. Causes of acute asthma attacks may be:

   A. intrinsic.
   B. extrinsic.
   C. chronic.
   D. All the above.

Correct answer is d.

10. Which of the following is an intrinsic cause of asthma?

   A. allergy to pollen.
   B. environmental contaminants.
   C. emotional stress.
   D. animal dander.

Correct answer is c.

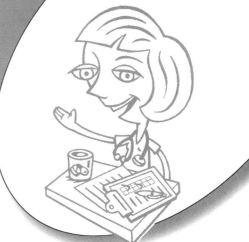

chapter 8

Rapid Sequence Intubation

LEARNING OBJECTIVES

At the end of this chapter, you will be able to:

1. Correctly identify the indications and contraindications for rapid sequence intubation.

2. Explain the appropriate selection of sedative agent and neuromuscular relaxant.

3. Understand the side effects and contraindications for use of the chosen medications.

4. Become familiar with the recommended equipment needed to safely complete a rapid sequence intubation.

5. Explain the differences between pediatric and adult RSI procedure.

KEY TERMS

Bradycardia
Fasciculations
Hyperkalemia
Increased intracranial pressure
Increased intraocular pressure
Malignant hyperthermia

Non-depolarizing neuromuscular
    blocking agents
Prolonged neuromuscular blockade
Rapid sequence induction
Rapid sequence intubation
Trismus

Introduction

Advanced airway management including rapid sequence intubation (RSI) is a fundamental component of advanced prehospital care. Securing airway patency and protection is an essential skill in caring for any respiratory compromised patient. It maximizes oxygenation of critically ill patients, enables their safe transport to hospital, and facilitates neuro-protection as well as rapid in-hospital investigation and definitive care. The extra time spent on scene securing an airway (even by skilled paramedics) is one of the greatest controversies in pre-hospital care. This time is often offset by the time saved during the transport and in-hospital phases of resuscitation as long as it is performed safely and expeditiously. Prehospital RSI scene times of less than 20 minutes are achievable and should be the target.

Prehospital RSI is potentially more risky than in-hospital RSI because of the difficulties of the prehospital environment, and therefore every effort must be made to ensure the safety of the procedure. In aviation and military settings it is well accepted, that the higher the acuity of the situation, the greater the need to remove individual procedural preference and the greater the need to adhere to a standard operating procedure.

Rapid Sequence Induction versus Rapid Sequence Intubation

Rapid sequence intubation (RSI) is a process where pharmacologic agents, specifically a sedative (ie, induction agent) and a neuromuscular blocking agent are administered in rapid succession to facilitate endotracheal intubation. RSI in the prehospital setting is usually conducted under less than optimal conditions and should be differentiated from RSI as practiced by anesthesiologists in a more controlled environment in the operating room to induce anesthesia in patients requiring intubation. RSI used to secure a definitive airway in the prehospital setting frequently involves uncooperative, non-fasted, unstable, critically ill patients. In anesthesia, the goal of RSI is to induce anesthesia while using a rapid sequence approach to decrease the possibility of aspiration.

With emergency RSI, the goal is to facilitate intubation with the additional benefit of decreasing the risk of aspiration. Although there are no randomized, controlled studies documenting the benefits of RSI, and there is controversy regarding various steps in RSI in adult and pediatric patients, RSI has become standard of care in emergency medicine airway treatment and has been advocated in airway management of intensive care unit or critically ill patients. RSI has also been used in the prehospital care setting, although the results have been mixed, especially in trauma patients (most notably in traumatic brain injury patients), such that an expert panel found that "the existing literature regarding paramedic RSI was in conclusive." Furthermore, training and experience "affect performance" and that a successful "paramedic RSI program is dependent on particular emergency medical services (EMS) and trauma system characteristics."[1-7]

[1]Wang HE, Davis DP, Wayne MA, et al. Prehospital rapid-sequence intubation—what does the evidence show? *Pre-hospital Emergency Care.* 2004; 8(4):366–377.

[2]Kovacs G, Law JA, Ross J, et al. Acute airway management in the emergency department by non-anesthesiologists. *Can J Anesthesia.* 2004;51(2):177–180.

[3]ACEP Policy Statement. Rapid-sequence intubation. Approved by ACEP Board of Directors—October 2006. Available at: www.ACEP.org Accessed 7/02/08.

[4]Walls RM. Rapid sequence intubation. In: Walls RM, Murphy MF, Luten RC, Succinylcholine Neider RE, eds. *Manual of emergency airway management.* Philadelphia: Lippincott Williams and Wilkins; 2004:22–32 [Chapter 3].

[5]Reynolds SF, Heffner J. Airway management of the critically ill patient. *Chest.* 2005;127(4):1397–412.

[6]Alves DW, Lawner B. Should RSI be performed in the prehospital setting? *Practical Summaries in Acute Care.* 2006;1(6):45–52.

[7]Davis DP, Fakhry SM, Wang HE, et al. Paramedic rapid sequence intubation for severe traumatic brain injury: perspectives from an expert panel. *Pre-hospital Emergency Care.* 2007;11(1):1–8.

Indications and Contraindications of RSI

Indications for RSI

As with all procedures, the decision to proceed with prehospital RSI must be based on an informed assessment of the risk of the procedure versus the clinical benefits.

The indications for prehospital emergency RSI are:

- Failure of airway patency
- Failure of airway protection
- Failure of ventilation or oxygenation
- Anticipated clinical course
- To facilitate safe transportation

    1. **Failure of airway patency.** Although simple airway maneuvers and adjuncts such as airway suctioning, chin-lift, oropharyngeal and nasopharyngeal airways may be essential initial measures to open and maintain a non-patent airway, these should be regarded as temporizing measures. Such patients will ALL require a secure airway at some point in their resuscitation and this should be considered in the prehospital phase provided it can be done safely and expeditiously.

    2. **Failure of airway protection.** An unconscious patient with an easily maintained airway and adequate ventilation is still at significant risk of passive regurgitation and aspiration of stomach contents, secretions or blood, particularly if transport times to hospital are prolonged. A patient with an unprotected airway is best defined by their inability to prevent aspiration of secretions, blood or vomitus and is indicated by an absence of spontaneous swallowing and/or failure to spontaneously clear blood, saliva or mucous from the oropharynx. Lack of a gag reflex or numerical assessment of Glasgow Coma Scale (GCS) (< 9) or motor scores (< 4) *cannot* be relied upon as an indicator of the need for intubation.

    3. **Failure of ventilation or oxygenation.** Patients with acute ventilatory failure or failure to maintain adequate oxygen saturation despite supplemental oxygen should be considered for prehospital emergency anesthesia and intubation. Such patients may have diminished respiratory drive due to head injury or critical chest injuries impairing ventilation.

    4. **Anticipated clinical course.** This indication refers to the patient who can be predicted to deteriorate (ie, head injuries, inhalational burns,

or spinal injuries) or where emergency anesthesia will be important in removing the work of breathing in the face of multiple major injuries. In the case of major trauma patients, whose management is certain to include a complex and potentially painful series of procedures and diagnostic evaluations as well as the operating theatre, early anesthesia and intubation should be considered.

5. **To facilitate safe transportation.** A subgroup of patients will require emergency anesthesia to ensure safe transportation particularly in rotary-winged or fixed-wing aircraft and/or where transport times are prolonged. These patients include agitated or uncooperative head-injured patients or those with severe psychiatric disturbance.

Contraindications of RSI
Absolute contraindications

- Total upper airway obstruction; requires surgical airway.
- Total loss of oropharyngeal/facial landmarks; requires surgical airway

Relative contraindications

- Anticipated "difficult" airway, in which endotracheal intubation may be unsuccessful, resulting in reliance on successful BVM ventilation.
- "Crash" airway is indicated for patient in cardiac arrest; immediate BVM ventilation, intubation or both should be performed without medications.

Advantages and Disadvantages of Rapid Sequence Intubation

The purpose of RSI is to make emergent intubation easier and safer, thereby increasing the success rate of intubation and decreasing the complications of intubation. The rationale behind RSI is to prevent aspiration and its potential problems (ie, aspiration pneumonia, increase in systemic arterial blood pressure, heart rate, plasma catecholamine release, intracranial pressure [ICP], and intra-ocular pressure [IOP]) that occur with endotracheal intubation. Blunting the rise in ICP may be critical in patients with impaired cerebral autoregulation from central nervous system illness/injury. Similarly, avoiding an increase in IOP may be desirable in the patient with glaucoma or an acute eye injury. RSI eliminates the normal protective airway reflexes (such as coughing, gagging, increased secretions, and laryngospasm) that can make intubation more diffi-cult. Use of RSI may limit cervical spine movement, thus, allowing for better control of the cervical spine during intubation with less potential for injury. RSI decreases trauma to the airway that occurs with intubation. RSI should also decrease or eliminate the discomfort that occurs with intubation and the patient's recall of the intubation.

Disadvantages of RSI are as follows:

1. The potential for side effects or complications related to the drugs administered for RSI

2. Prolonged intubation leading to hypoxia, and;

3. "Emergent" or a "crash" airway resulting in a cricothyroidotomy or other "emergent" airway procedure.

Rapid Sequence Intubation: "THE PROCEDURE"

Rapid sequence intubation generally consists of seven steps. These seven steps can be modified when appropriate to fit a specific clinical situation. "The seven Ps of RSI" are as follows:

1. Preparation and patient positioning

2. Preoxygenation

3. Pretreatment

4. Paralysis with induction

5. Protection and positioning of the airway

6. Placement of the endotracheal tube in the trachea

7. Postintubation management and patient packaging

Step 1—Preparation and Patient Positioning

Preparation involves having all the necessary equipment and supplies including medications that may be needed for an emergency intubation. This equipment includes oxygen, suction, bag-valve mask (BVM), laryngoscope and blades, endotracheal (ET) tubes with a stylet with one size larger and smaller than the anticipated ET size, resuscitation equipment, and supplies for rescue maneuvers (ie, laryngeal mask airways [LMA] or cricothyrotomy) in case of a failed intubation. The patient should have an intravenous line placed and be put on continuous monitoring to include vital signs (heart rate, respirations, blood pressure, pulse oximetry), cardiac rhythm monitoring, and, preferably, capnography. The mnemonic Suction, Oxygen, Airway, Pharmacology, Monitoring, and Equipment (SOAPME) is one way to remember the essential equipment needed for intubation. For the airway, include the ET tubes, laryngoscopes, blades, stylets, and BVM. For pharmacology, select, draw up, and label the appropriate medications (sedative, neuromuscular blocker, ancillary drugs) based on the history, physical examination, and equipment available.

Assembling adequate personnel needed to assist in the procedure and assigning their roles is also a key component of the preparation phase. Patient assessment should be done at this time. A thorough history and physical examination should be done to identify any condition, illnesses, or injuries that may negatively affect airway procedures/manipulations, medication administration, BVM ventilation, intubation, RSI, or rescue airway procedures.

The preparation step is used to monitor, assemble, patient (MAP) assessment out a treatment plan for intubation using RSI and a back up contingency plan in case of a failed intubation (can't ventilate, can't intubate scenario).

Step 2—Preoxygenation

Preoxygenation should be occurring during the preparation step. The purpose of preoxygenation is to replace the nitrogen in the patient's functional residual capacity (FRC) with oxygen or "nitrogen wash-out oxygen wash-in." "Denitrogenation" can be accomplished in 3 to 5 minutes by having the patient breathe 100% oxygen via a tight-fitting facemask or, if time is an issue, with four vital capacity breaths. Depending on circumstances, as long a period of preoxygenation as possible, (up to 5 minutes) should be administered. Ideally, positive pressure ventilation should be avoided during the preoxygenation step because of a risk for gastric insufflation and possible regurgitation. Because effective ventilation by the patient is not feasible in many prehospital patients, BVM ventilation may be necessary in apneic patients or patients with ineffective spontaneous breathing. In the preoxygenation phase, replacing the nitrogen reservoir in the lungs with oxygen allows 3 to 5 minutes of apnea without significant hypoxemia in the normoxic adult. One caveat to remember is that certain patients have a lesser FRC (ie, infants, children, and patients with an elevated diaphragm, specifically obese adults or pregnant women). These patients will become hypoxic in a shorter time, ie, a normal child or an obese adult may start to desaturate within 2 minutes, while a normal adult may tolerate up to 5 minutes of apnea before they become significantly hypoxic.

Step 3—Pretreatment

Ancillary medications are administered during the pretreatment step to mitigate the negative physiologic responses to intubation. For maximal efficacy, the pretreatment drugs should precede the induction agent by 3 minutes, although this is not always possible. The pretreatment phase and preoxygenation phase can (and usually) do occur simultaneously during most instances of RSI in the prehospital setting. Medications and their usual dosages that may be given during the pretreatment phase are lidocaine 1.0 to 1.5 mg/kg, fentanyl 2 to 3 µg/kg, and atropine 0.02 mg/kg (minimum 0.1 mg, maximum 0.5 mg).

What Went Wrong?   The clinical indications for pretreatment drugs are: (1) for patients with elevated ICP and impaired autoregulation administer lidocaine and fentanyl, (2) patients with major vessel dissection or rupture or those with significant ischemic heart disease give fentanyl, (3) adults with significant reactive airway disease, premedicate with lidocaine, and (4) atropine is indicated for pediatric patients < 10-year-olds and in patients with significant bradycardia if succinylcholine is given. One caveat to remember is to give fentanyl with caution to any patient in shock (whether compensated or uncompensated) who is dependent on sympathetic drive because of a potential decrease in blood pressure with fentanyl administration.

In patients who are receiving succinylcholine as their induction agent and who are at risk for increased ICP, one-tenth of the normal paralyzing dose of a non-depolarizing (ND) neuromuscular blocking agent (NMB) can be given 3 minutes before receiving succinylcholine. The purpose of the defasciculating dose of the ND-NMB is to prevent the fasciculations (and therefore, the increase in ICP) that occurs with succinylcholine. For example, the dose would be 10% of the paralyzing dose of rocuronium (10% of 0.6 mg/kg is 0.06 mg/kg). The mnemonic "LOAD" has been used to indicate the pretreatment drugs for RSI (Figure 8-1).

Step 4—Paralysis with Induction

Paralysis with induction is achieved by the rapid intravenous administration in quick succession of the induction agent and the NMB. The selection of a specific sedative depends on multiple factors:

1. The clinical scenario, which includes patient factors (includes cardiorespiratory and neurologic status, allergies, comorbidity).

2. The paramedic's experience/training.

3. Prehospital factors

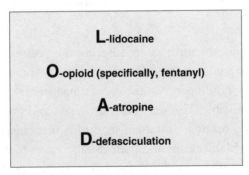

L-lidocaine

O-opioid (specifically, fentanyl)

A-atropine

D-defasciculation

FIGURE 8-1 • **LOAD**-pretreatment drugs for RSI.

TABLE 8-1 Clinical Actions of RSI Sedative/Induction Agents

Sedative	Dose	Induction Time	B/P Effect	ICP Effect	Comments
Thiopental	3-5 mg/kg	10-15 seconds	Lowers	Lowers	Bronchospasm, avoid in porphyria
Etomidate	0.3 mg/kg	30-45 seconds	Neutral	Lowers	Adrenal suppression, possible epileptogenic
Propofol	1-2 mg/kg	10-15 seconds	Lowers	Lowers	Maintenance sedation infusion
Ketamine	1-2 mg/kg	30-45 seconds	Raises	Raises	Bronchodilation
Fentanyl	1-2 µg/kg	30-45 seconds	Neutral	Possibly lowers	Chest wall rigidity
Midazolam	0.1-0.3 mg/kg	120-180 seconds	Neutral or lowers with higher doses	Neutral	Long onset, amnesia

4. Characteristics of the sedative. Sedatives commonly used for induction during RSI are barbiturates (pentobarbitol, thiopental, and methohexitol), opioids (fentanyl), dissociative anesthetics (ketamine), and non-barbiturate sedatives (etomidate, propofol, and the benzodiazepines). The dosages and characteristics of these agents and are summarized in Table 8-1. One caveat to remember is that the induction dosages of these sedatives may be different (generally, slightly higher) than the dose used for sedation. For example, for etomidate the usual dose for procedural sedation is 0.2 mg/kg and for RSI is 0.3 mg/kg.

Step 5—Protection and Positioning

Positioning of the head and neck is essential to achieve the best view of the glottic opening for conventional laryngoscopy. This is performed by aligning the three axis: oral, pharyngeal, and laryngeal. This can be achieved by extension and elevation of the neck to obtain the "sniffing position"; assuming there are no contraindications such as known or potential cervical spine injury (Figure 8-2). Protection refers to the use of maneuvers to prevent regurgitation of gastric contents with possible aspiration.

Cricoid pressure and the controversy behind the maneuver

- There is no evidence that even well-applied cricoid pressure (Sellick's maneuver) prevents passive aspiration. It is most commonly poorly performed.

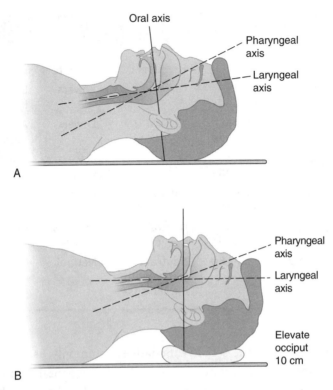

FIGURE 8-2 • Axis alignment.
Reproduced with permission from Tintinalli JE, Stapczynski JS, Cline DM, Ma OJ, Cydulka RK, Meckler GD, eds. *Tintinalli's Emergency Medicine: A Comprehensive Study Guide.* 7th ed. 2011. New York: Copyright © McGraw-Hill Education. All rights reserved.

There is an evidence that cricoid pressure may reduce tone at the lower esophageal sphincter, significantly impair laryngoscopic view and cause unwanted movements of the cervical spine. It should no longer be routinely applied to patients undergoing prehospital RSI. If the paramedic decides to use cricoid pressure for the RSI they must ensure the cricoid operator is briefed appropriately and cricoid pressure removed if laryngoscopic view is difficult.

- External laryngeal manipulation (ELM) has been demonstrated to improve laryngoscopic view and should be used whenever initial view is suboptimal. The paramedic manipulates the thyroid cartilage to maximize their view and an assistant can be directed to hold the thyroid cartilage in position during intubation. It is important to recognize the difference between this technique, cricoid pressure, and B.U.R.P.

- The uncleared C-spine should be routinely protected in all blunt trauma patients and this should be performed by an assistant holding the head from the left side of the patient. The cervical collar should be open and the mandible free of any restrictions for intubation.

- In many patients, the cervical collar causes significant neck extension and this is exaggerated in those with a large body habitus. This can be corrected by placing a folded towel or SAM splint beneath the occiput to maintain a neutral head position. This may reduce the tendency of the paramedic to "suspend" the head from the laryngoscope and flex the neck. If cervical spine precautions are not needed (ie, burns patients or following submersion incidents) the patient should be positioned in the "ear to sternal notch position" (ESP) which greatly improves laryngoscopic view.

Step 6—Placement of the Endotracheal Tube in the Trachea

When the jaw becomes flaccid from the paralytics, it is time to begin intubation by standard methods. ET tube placement should be confirmed by the usual techniques; direct visualization, auscultation, absent epigastric sounds, and waveform $EtCO_2$.

Step 7—Postintubation Management and Patient Packaging

After ET tube placement and confirmation, the ET tube must be secured. Use a commercial tube holder to secure the ET in place. Waveform capnography is the gold standard of care postintubation and should be used for every intubated patient. To reduce the possibility of dislodgement or right stem placement of the ET during patient movement, the use of cervical collar in medical as well as trauma patients significantly reduces hyperflexion and/or hyperextension of the neck during patient movement. In hospital, a chest radiograph is done not only to check for proper ET tube placement but also to evaluate the pulmonary status and to monitor for any complications of the intubation and RSI. Continued sedation and analgesia, sometimes with paralysis as well as cardiopulmonary monitoring, is indicated as long as the patient requires advanced airway support.

Pharmacology: Sedative Agents for Rapid Sequence Intubation

According to the National Emergency Airway Registry (NEAR) study, the most frequently used induction agents were etomidate (69%), midazolam (16%), fentanyl (6%), and ketamine (3%). Considering just pediatric patients using the NEAR etomidate was the most commonly used induction agent but was used in less than half the patients (only 42% compared with 69% for all patients), followed by thiopental (22%), midazolam (18%), and ketamine (7%).

Etomidate

Etomidate, the most commonly used sedative for RSI in adults, can also be administered for pediatric RSI. The usual dose is 0.3 mg/kg or 20 mg in a 70-kg adult. It often is used in trauma patients with known or potential bleeding, hypovolemic patients, and patients with limited cardiac reserve, because it does not have significant cardiovascular effects. Etomidate also decreases ICP and the cerebral metabolic rate, which suggests that it may have a neuroprotective effect. These features are why some medical directors consider it the sedative of choice in patients who have multiple trauma, with both a head injury and hemorrhage or shock. Etomidate does inhibit 11-beta-hydroxylase, an enzyme necessary for adrenal steroid production. Transient adrenal suppression has been noted after a single dose of etomidate, although this is probably not clinically significant. There are data that indicate that etomidate has a negative impact on patient outcome in critically ill patients with sepsis and septic shock. This has led to the suggestion that a corticosteroid be co-administered when etomidate is given for RSI. Although either dexamethasone (0.1 mg/kg) or hydrocortisone (1-2 mg/kg) may be given, dexamethasone often is chosen because it does not interfere with the adrenocorticotropin hormone (ACTH) stimulation test, which may be needed to later test for adrenal insufficiency. In any case, infusions of etomidate for continued postintubation sedation are contraindicated. Myoclonus is another side effect of etomidate that may interfere with intubation if a paralytic is not used, although this is not the situation with RSI in which a sedative and paralytic generally are co-administered in quick succession.

Barbiturates

Thiopental is the most commonly used barbiturate for pediatric RSI and may be the most commonly used barbiturate for anesthesia induction. However, it is used less commonly than etomidate for prehospital or emergency department (ED) RSI, at least partly because many prehospital and ED RSI patients are hemodynamically unstable. Thiopental decreases both cerebral blood flow and the metabolic demands of the brain, which makes it an ideal sedative agent in patients with known increased ICP or patients with head injury who are hemodynamically stable. Thiopental has negative cardiovascular effects: myocardial depression and peripheral vasodilatation. Thus, hypotension with associated hypoperfusion can occur in patients who are hypovolemic or have myocardial depression. Generally, when hypotension occurs, there is a compensatory baroreceptor mediated reflex tachycardia. Unfortunately, patients who are hypovolemic or in shock or who are already tachycardic may not be capable of further compensatory heart rate increases and can experience a drop in blood pressure with thiopental administration. Similarly, patients with preexisting cardiovascular disease may also experience hypotension when given thiopental.

The conclusion is to avoid using thiopental, if possible, in patients with underlying cardiovascular disease, hypovolemia, or shock. Or limit thiopental to small frequent doses (1-3 mg/kg) while carefully monitoring blood pressure.

Thiopental also has some respiratory side effects. It has a dose- and rate-related (ie, high dose, rapid administration) respiratory depression of the central nervous system (CNS) that can cause apnea, especially in head injured or hypovolemic patients. With "light" anesthesia, several untoward effects may occur, especially during airway manipulation: catecholamine release causing systemic or intracranial hypertension, laryngospasm, cough, and bronchospasm, especially in asthmatic patients. To mitigate or avoid these negative effects, it has been recommended to co-administer an analgesic (such as fentanyl) especially in head-injured patients. Tissue necrosis can occur with intra-arterial injection or extravasation, so it is critical that thiopental be given intravenously as a dilute solution while being careful to avoid any tissue infiltration.

Ketamine

Ketamine, a dissociative anesthetic, exerts its effects by interrupting the connection between the thalamo-neocortical tracts and the limbic system. Unlike all the other sedatives, it has an additional advantage in that it also has analgesic properties. Ketamine's sympathomimetic effects, acting via a centrally mediated mechanism, cause an increase in heart rate, blood pressure, and cardiac output. This makes ketamine an excellent sedative in patients who are hypotensive, especially if secondary to shock, hemorrhage, dehydration, pericarditis, or tamponade. However, these sympathomimetic effects are undesirable in patients who already have significant hypertension or tachycardia.

Ketamine also causes an increase in ICP by both an increase in systemic blood pressure and cerebral vasodilatation. Therefore, ketamine is contraindicated in patients with ICP, intracerebral hemorrhage, intracranial mass or head trauma; although a recent study has challenged this contraindication. One French study compared the cerebral hemodynamics of ketamine combined with midazolam and found no significant difference in ICP or cerebral perfusion pressure when compared with midazolam sufentanil. It has previously been thought that young age (ie, < 6 months) was a contraindication to the use of ketamine. However, a recent study indicates that ketamine is safe and effective even in neonates. Ketamine is probably the sedative of choice for asthmatic patients for many reasons. Ketamine, through the release of endogenous catecholamines, relieves bronchospasm by dilating bronchial smooth muscle and stimulating the pulmonary beta receptors. Ketamine increases tracheobronchial/oropharyngeal secretions. This may have a positive effect by decreasing mucus plugging in some cases. The excess secretions may, however, interfere with visualization of the airway during laryngoscopy. Fortunately pretreatment with atropine (preferred for RSI) can reduce secretions. The dose of atropine for RSI is 0.01 to 0.02 mg/kg intravenously with a minimum of 0.1 mg and a maximum of 0.5 to 1.0 mg. Although the routine use of atropine has been questioned, the consensus is that it is still useful in selected patients. Atropine is used for RSI because it causes an increase in heart rate, which is desirable when offsetting the bradycardic effects of succinylcholine during RSI.

Ketamine has respiratory/cardiovascular stability and maintains airway reflexes. As with all sedatives, rare instances of apnea and laryngospasm have been reported. Ketamine, an analog of phencyclidine (PCP), is associated with an occasional emergence reaction, so its use should probably be avoided in psychotic patients. Small doses of midazolam have been given for the treatment of emergence reactions. Traditional teaching is that co-administration of a benzodiazepam (ie, midazolam) with ketamine will prevent emergence reactions. This teaching has been challenged recently by several studies that reported the prophylactic administration of benzodiazepine did not decrease the incidence of emergence reactions but actually increased the risk of respiratory depression and prolonged recovery, while paradoxically increasing the incidence of emergence reactions in a subset of patients.

Benzodiazepines

Midazolam is the most commonly used benzodiazepine for RSI and prehospital sedation primarily because it has a rapid onset and short duration. Other advantages of midazolam versus diazepam include fewer adverse effects, better amnesia, and greater potency. All of the benzodiazepines, including midazolam, diazepam, and lorazepam, have sedative, hypnotic, amnestic, anxiolytic, muscle relaxant, and anticonvulsant properties. Benzodiazepines bind to a specific benzodiazepine receptor site on the gamma-aminobutyric acid (GABA) receptor. GABA is an inhibitory neurotransmitter. This opens a chloride channel causing hyperpolarization of the neuronal cell membrane, thereby blocking neuronal depolarization or activation. The antagonist, flumazenil, can reverse the effects of the benzodiazepines. Advantages of the benzodiazepines include minimal cardiovascular effects (unless the patient is hypovolemic), can be used in patients with coronary artery disease, positive nitroglycerin-like effect in patients with heart failure (decreases the increased ventricular filling pressure), and seizure treatment. The main disadvantage of the benzodiazepines is that they can cause respiratory depression and apnea. Other uncommon side effects are paradoxical agitation, vomiting, coughing, and hiccups. The benzodiazepine dosage for RSI and sedation varies widely and should be decreased when given along with opioids, in the elderly, patients with renal failure, or severe hepatic disease, or significant heart disease.

Propofol

Propofol is an ultra-short-acting sedative hypnotic agent. It has no analgesic effects, and its amnestic effects are variable. The advantages of propofol are its very quick onset and short duration. It also has antiemetic properties, can be used in malignant hyperthermia patients, and the dosage is unchanged for patients with renal or liver disease, although higher doses may be needed in pediatric patients and lower doses in geriatric patients. Side effects include hypotension, bradycardia, hypoxia and apnea, so it should be administered slowly. Propofol also has negative cardiovascular effects so it should be used with caution in patients with volume depletion, hypotension, or cardiovascular disease. Because of these side effects/complications its use as a sedative for RSI is limited in many prehospital patients.

Pathophysiology

A discussion of the anatomy and physiology of the neuromuscular junction is valuable in understanding how the neuromuscular blockers work.

Anatomy

The neuromuscular or myoneural junction is the junction between the nerve fiber ending or nerve terminal, the muscle fiber including the muscle fiber membrane or sarcolemma, and the interposed synaptic cleft (synaptic space). The motor end plate refers to the complex of branching nerve terminals that in vaginate into (but actually lie outside) the sarcolemma. Subneural clefts are folds of the muscle cell (myocyte) membrane, which markedly increase the surface area at which the synaptic neurotransmitter acetylcholine (ACh) can act. A single terminal branch of the nerve axon lies in the synaptic gutter or synaptic trough, which is an invagination of the sarcolemma. Structures found in the nerve terminal include synaptic vesicles containing the neurotransmitter ACh, the dense bar areas (ACh from the vesicles is released into the synaptic cleft through the neural membrane adjacent to the densebars), voltage gated calcium channels (which are protein particles that penetrate the neural membrane), and mitochondria (which supply the adenosine triphosphate [ATP] that acts as the energy source for the synthesis of ACh).

The nicotinic receptor, a protein particle located on the postsynaptic myocyte membrane has two parts: a binding component and an ionophore component. The binding component projects outward from the postsynaptic myocyte membrane into the synaptic space where it binds the neurotransmitter ACh. The ionosphere component extends through the postsynaptic neural membrane to the interior of the postsynaptic membrane. The ionosphere may serve as an ion channel that permits the movement of ions (in this case primarily sodium ions, as well as other ions) through the membrane.

Neurotransmitter: Acetylcholine

Acetylcholine, the neurotransmitter at cholinergic synapses, is released from the ending of preganglionic and postganglionic parasympathetic nerves and preganglionic sympathetic nerves. ACh is synthesized from choline and acetic acid in the nerve and packaged in vesicles. With nerve stimulation, the impulse reaches the nerve ending causing the ACh vesicles to travel to the nerve surface and rupture, thereby releasing ACh into the synaptic space (synaptic cleft). Exocytosis is the process whereby the ACh containing vesicles fuse with the nerve terminal membrane and release their ACh. When the action potential depolarizes the presynaptic membranes, the calcium ion channels open, increasing the neural membrane permeability to calcium, allowing calcium ions to stream into the presynaptic nerve ending. The calcium ions bind with "release sites" that are unique protein molecules on the inner surface of the presynaptic neural membranes. The coupling of the calcium ion to the specific protein molecule opens the release sites, which permits the vesicles to release the neurotransmitter ACh into the synaptic space. ACh then diffuses across the synaptic cleft to the motor endplate. Attachment of ACh to the nicotinic receptors on the skeletal muscle leads to a conformational change in the nicotinic receptor. This altered protein molecule on the nicotinic skeletal muscle receptor increases the permeability of the skeletal myocyte cell to various ions (sodium, potassium, chloride, and calcium) with an influx of sodium into the skeletal myocyte. This produces a large positive potential charge within the skeletal.

The flow of ions and the action potential physiologically, an abrupt increase of greater than 20 to 30 millivolts causes further opening of additional sodium channels, allowing for an action potential in the skeletal muscle fiber membrane. A weak local end plate potential, less than 20 to 30 millivolts, will be insufficient to cause an action potential in the skeletal muscle fiber membrane. This is what happens with various drugs or toxins. For example, the drug curare competes with ACh for the nicotinic receptor sites on the skeletal muscle, which results in blocking the action of ACh in opening the sodium ion channels. The botulinum toxin prevents depolarization by decreasing the amount of ACh released by the nerve terminals. The flow of ions is important, because decreasing the resting membrane potential voltage to a less negative value increases neural excitability leading to depolarization when the threshold (about 50 millivolts in skeletal muscle) is reached, whereas conversely increasing the resting membrane potential to a more negative number makes the neuron less excitable.

Neuromuscular Blockers

Neuromuscular blocking agents (NMBs) are substances that paralyze skeletal muscles by blocking nerve impulse transmission at the neuromuscular or myoneural (muscle-nerve) junction. There are several critical factors to remember with RSI. First, a sedative is co-administered with the NMB. Patients given an NMB may be aware of their environment, including painful stimuli, even though they are unable to respond. Failure to sedate the patient allows the possibility of negative physiologic responses to airway manipulation such as increased ICP, hypertension, and tachycardia. In addition, the patient may be aware of and remember the intubation, which is considered inhumane. Concomitant sedative use limits or helps avoid these adverse physiologic responses to airway manipulation and may even result in a better view of the airway during laryngoscopy.

However, whenever an NMB is used, the paramedic must be prepared for a difficult or failed airway with the possibility that a surgical airway may be necessary if the patient cannot be oxygenated or ventilated adequately with a bag-valve mask or extra glottic device. Assessment of the airway, especially if there is the potential for a difficult or failed airway, should be done before administering an NMB. NMBs are depolarizing or non-depolarizing. Depolarizing agents mimic the action of ACh. They cause a sustained depolarization of the neuromuscular junction, which prevents muscle contraction. Non-depolarizing agents work by competitive inhibition to block ACh's action at the neuromuscular junction to prevent depolarization. According to the NEAR, the most frequently used NMBs were succinylcholine (82%), rocuronium (12%), and vecuronium (5%). For pediatric patients only, succinylcholine (90%) was also the most commonly used NMB, with vecuronium used in7%, and rocuronium in 2%.

Pharmacology

All NMBs are structurally similar to the neurotransmitter ACh. ACh and all NMBs are quaternary ammonium compounds; the positive charges of these compounds at the nitrogen atom, account for their attraction to the cholinergic nicotinic (inotropic) receptors at the neuromuscular junction and at other nicotinic receptor sites throughout the body. This nonspecific action at sites throughout the body, ie, nicotinic (ganglionic) and muscarinic autonomic sites, not just at the neuromuscular junction, helps explain some of their side effects.

Depolarizing Neuromuscular Blocking Agents

Succinylcholine

Since 1952, succinylcholine has been the only depolarizing agent available in the United States. It has been used in countless patients since its introduction as an NMB. It is the most commonly used NMB for prehospital and ED RSI. Succinylcholine is the prototype of the depolarizing agents. Because its chemical structure (ie, quaternary ammonium compound) is similar to that of ACh, it binds to the acetylcholine receptor on the motor end plate and depolarizes the postjunctional neuro muscular membrane, resulting in continuous stimulation of the motor end plate ACh receptors. The neuromuscular block/motor paralysis is terminated when the NMB (ie, succinylcholine) unbinds from the ACh receptor and diffuses back into the circulation where it is hydrolyzed by plasma cholinesterase. Plasma cholinesterase (also referred to as "pseudocholinesterase" or "butylcholinesterase") rapidly hydrolyses succinylcholine to succinylmonocholine (a very weak NMB) and choline. Succinylcholine's short duration of action is caused by the rapid hydrolysis by plasma cholinesterase both before succinylcholine reaches and after succinylcholine leaves the neuromuscular junction, because there is minimal if any pseudocholinesterase at the neuromuscular junction. Some ACh may diffuse back into the nerve terminal, although the majority of ACh is hydrolyzed by plasma cholinesterase. Muscle contraction will not reoccur until the neuromuscular junction returns to the resting state and then is depolarized again. Transient fasciculations (caused by initial depolarization) are followed by blockade of neuromuscular transmission with motor paralysis when succinylcholine is administered.

The major advantages of succinylcholine are its rapid onset with complete motor paralysis occurring within 45 to 60 seconds and short duration of action lasting only 6 to 10 minutes when given in the recommended 1.5-mg/kg intravenous dose.

Dosing of Succinylcholine

There are some "PEARLS" regarding succinylcholine dosing. Use the total body weight (not the lean weight) even in the morbidly obese or pregnant patient. Do not underdose the drug. It is preferable to overestimate rather than underestimate the dose because an insufficient dose may make it difficult to intubate if the patient is not adequately paralyzed. Thus, the preferred dose is 1.5 mg/kg (or about 100 mg in a 70-kg adult) (some suggest 1.5-2.0 mg/kg in an adult) and not 1 mg/kg as stated in some references. The recommended succinylcholine dose in infants (including neonates) is 2 mg/kg based on their higher volume of distribution, and some even recommend up to 3 mg/kg in newborns. Administer succinylcholine as a rapid bolus followed by a 20 to 30 cc saline flush to avoid incomplete paralysis. Succinylcholine has also been given intramuscularly in a 3 to 4-mg/kg dose in a rare life-threatening situation in which there is inability to obtain venous access. Repeat doses or prolonged use of succinylcholine is to be avoided for several reasons. Repeat dosing or prolonged use of succinylcholine potentiates its effects at the sympathetic ganglia and vagal effects. The negative muscarinic effects from vagal stimulation may lead to bradycardia and hypotension even at recommended doses. This is one reason some experts recommend atropine pretreatment in infants/small children, anyone with significant bradycardia, and those receiving multiple doses of succinylcholine. Desensitization blockage, whereby the neuromuscular membrane returns to the resting state and becomes resistant to further depolarization with succinylcholine can also occur with repeat doses of succinylcholine. In patients with myasthenia gravis, there is a functional decrease in ACh receptors at the neuromuscular junction secondary to an antibody-mediated autoimmune destruction of the ACh receptors. Succinylcholine can be used in patients with myasthenia gravis, although the dose is increased to 2 mg/kg to reach and activate the remaining ACh receptors unaffected by the disease.

Be careful to check the expiration date on the drug vial, especially if the drug is not refrigerated, because succinylcholine degrades gradually at room temperature. Refrigeration lowers the drug's degradation rate so that it maintains 90% activity for up to 90 days.

Contraindications

The absolute contraindications to succinylcholine are: (1) a history of malignant hyperthermia in the patient or family, and (2) patients at high risk of severe hyperkalemia.

Side Effects of Succinylcholine

Malignant hyperthermia   Malignant hyperthermia is a rare genetic myopathetic disorder precipitated by multiple drugs, especially certain inhalational anesthetics (such as halothane, sevoflurane, desiflurane, isoflurane) and succinylcholine. It is thought to be caused by an abnormal ryanodine receptor causing marked leakage of calcium from the sarcoplasmic reticulum of skeletal muscle cells resulting in extremely high intracellular calcium levels. Symptoms generally begin within an hour of the drug or anesthetic administration but may be delayed for hours. The clinical presentation generally includes muscle rigidity (especially masseter stiffness), increased CO_2 production, acidosis, sympathetic hyperactivity with hyperthermia (up to 113°F), and sinus tachycardia.

Complications that can occur include rhabdomyolysis, electrolyte abnormalities, dysrhythmias, hypotension/shock, disseminated intravascular coagulation, and death. With intensive medical therapy including dantrolene sodium, the mortality rate has decreased from 70% to less than 10%. Thus, any history of malignant hyperthermia in the patient or any family member is an absolute contraindication to succinylcholine. Unfortunately, with RSI in the prehospital setting, a history is often not available.

Hyperkalemia   Even in "normal" patients, succinylcholine may increase the serum potassium up to 0.5 mEq/L because of depolarization of the myocytes (skeletal muscle cells). Generally, the rise has no clinical significance except in patients with a predisposition to hyperkalemia, such as a patient with rhabdomyolysis or patients with chronic skeletal muscle disease in whom there is "up-regulation" from increased sensitization of extra junctional ACh receptor in muscle. Such susceptibility is not present immediately after the onset of neuromuscular disease or after a traumatic injury but can develop within 4 to 5 days and last indefinitely.

Hyperkalemia can occur whenever there is massive tissue destruction or severe muscular wasting. The extra junctional ACh receptor sensitization becomes clinically significant 4 to 5 days after injury or illness onset, so the risk of life-threatening hyperkalemia does not start until days (usually 3-5 days) after the injury or illness onset. This is important because succinylcholine can be used in the acute trauma patient, the acute stroke or head injured patient, or a patient with neuromuscular disease, immediately after their injury or disease onset. Patients with extensive muscle wasting from denervating neuromuscular diseases include patients with a spinal cord injury, multiple sclerosis, motor neuron injury, stroke, and muscular dystrophies (ie, Duchene muscular dystrophy or Becker muscular dystrophy). With rhabdomyolysis, the destruction of myocytes secondary to tissue injury releases potassium from the cells causing the serum potassium level to increase. The second mechanism, up-regulation, causes hyperkalemia because the abnormal upregulated ACh receptor s have low conductance and prolonged ion channel opening times that lead to an increase in potassium. Up-regulation usually occurs within 3 to 5 days and lasts indefinitely, even years (3 or more years) after an acute injury or a progressive disease. Giving defasciculating doses of nonpolarizing NMBAs does not affect the hyperkalemic response. The hyperkalemic response to succinylcholine has also been reported in patients in the intensive care unit with life-threatening infections, especially if there is atrophy and chemical denervation of the ACh receptors.

Although the longstanding tenet has been to avoid succinylcholine in patients in chronic renal failure who have normokalemia, there is no supportive evidence for this. In reality, most patients with renal failure undergo successful RSI with succinylcholine without any untoward cardiovascular events. However, succinylcholine is not recommended for patients with known hyperkalemia because of concern that even the "usual" potassium increase of 0.5 mEq/L may precipitate fatal dysrhythmias in a patient with existing significant hyperkalemia and acidosis. Thus, succinylcholine should be avoided in patients with ECG changes of hyperkalemia.

Bradycardia   Bradycardia after succinylcholine administration most frequently occurs in infants and children because of the vagal predominance of their autonomic nervous system, but can also occur in patients of any age with repeated succinylcholine doses. Pretreatment with atropine, 0.02 mg/kg, minimizes or eliminates this bradycardia response.

Prolonged neuromuscular blockade   Any factor that inhibits the breakdown of succinylcholine will prolong neuromuscular blockade and paralysis. An abnormal form or a decrease in pseudocholinesterase (either acquired or congenital) leads to prolonged paralysis from delayed degradation of succinylcholine. Various genetic variants of pseudocholinesterase exist including one disorder with defective pseudocholinesterase in which individuals receiving succinylcholine remain paralyzed for up to 6 to 8 hours after a single dose of succinylcholine. Decreased pseudocholinesterase levels can also occur secondary to various acquired disorders such as liver disease, renal failure, anemia, pregnancy, chronic cocaine use, increased age, connective tissue disease, various malignancies, and organophosphate poisoning. However, this finding has little clinical significance because even large decreases in pseudocholinesterase activity cause small increments in the duration of neuromuscular paralysis after succinylcholine administration because baseline pseudocholinesterase levels are quite high.

Increased intracranial pressure   The effect of succinylcholine on ICP has been debated with various studies noting conflicting results. Some researchers have noted small increases in ICP (range, 5-10 mm Hg), whereas other studies have shown no increase. More importantly, there has been no evidence of neurologic deterioration secondary to the transient ICP increase associated with succinylcholine.

Pretreatment with a non-depolarizing NMB prevents the increase in ICP, although the additional time and steps associated with such pretreatment may be impractical and time consuming in an airway emergency, and the suggested pretreatment dose of a non-depolarizing NMB may, by itself, cause incomplete paralysis. The extensive experience with succinylcholine in the clinical setting of patients with acute intracerebral pathology documenting its safety and efficacy coupled with the dangers of a failed airway with secondary cerebral insult from hypoxia obviates against these theoretical, small, and likely clinically insignificant transient increases in ICP with succinylcholine.

Increased intraocular pressure   Succinylcholine can increase IOP by 6 to 8 mm Hg. Succinylcholine has been used safely and effectively in patients with penetrating eye injuries during RSI anesthesia. Some experts have recommended the use of succinylcholine even in patients with an open globe injury if there is a need for emergent securing of the airway, citing the greater risk from allowing the negative side effects of an uncontrolled intubation (including hypoxia and coughing or vomiting, which also likely results in a greater increase in IOP.)

Trismus   Masseter muscle spasm (trismus) occurs in 0.001% to 0.1% of patients after succinylcholine administration. It has been associated with malignant hyperthermia. However, it may occur in isolation. Treatment includes giving a standard dose of a ND-NMB, although a cricothyrotomy has been necessary in rare cases.

Fasciculations   Fasciculations are involuntary, unsynchronized muscle contractions. They are caused by the depolarization of ACh receptors. This, in turn, initiates an action potential, which is propagated to all of the muscles supplied by the nerve. Fasciculations have various negative effects: myalgias, increased creatinine kinase, myoglobinemia, increased catecholamines (with secondary increased blood pressure and heart rate), and increased cardiac output (increased oxygen consumption and increased carbon dioxide production). The transient small increases in cerebral blood flow and ICP that occur with succinylcholine may be caused by fasciculations. Defasciculation can be accomplished by pretreatment with lidocaine at 1.5 mg/kg or 10% of the intubating dose of a non-depolarizing NMB.

Non-depolarizing Neuromuscular Blocking Agents

Non-depolarizing (ND) NMBs competitively block ACh transmission at the postjunctional cholinergic nicotinic receptors. Unlike succinylcholine, which causes a conformational change in the ACh receptor resulting in depolarization of the neuromuscular junction, the non-depolarizing NMB prevents ACh from access to the nicotinic receptor, thereby preventing muscle contraction. Fasciculations do not occur with the ND-NMBs. Some ultra-short ND NMBs are undergoing research, but they are not yet clinically available. As stated earlier in the chapter, the only ultra-short NMB available in the United States is the depolarizing NMB, succinylcholine. However, doubling the dose of rocuronium from 0.6 mg/kg to 1.2 mg/kg shortens the onset of complete neuromuscular blockade from about 1.5 minutes (mean, 89 seconds) to 1 minute (mean, 55 seconds). If succinylcholine cannot be used and intubation in less than 90 seconds is needed, then the higher doses of the ND-NMB can be used. The high dose regimen for RSI is preferred over the "priming technique," whereby a small subparalyzing dose of the ND-NMB (ie, 10% of the intubating dose) is given 2 to 4 minutes before the second large dose for tracheal intubation for several reasons: intubating conditions are less optimal than with succinylcholine, priming has risks (including aspiration), and there are side effects.

Indications for Non-depolarizing Neuromuscular Blocking Agents

The ND-NMBs are used:

1. For muscle relaxation if succinylcholine is contraindicated or unavailable.

2. To maintain postintubation paralysis (remember that repeated doses of succinylcholine should be avoided, if possible).

3. As a pretreatment agent to lessen or eliminate the fasciculations and their side effects (ie, myalgia's and increased IOP, ICP, intragastric pressure [IGP]) associated with succinylcholine use. The contraindication for the use of ND-NMBs is the same as for a depolarizing NMB, inability to secure the airway with the possibility of a difficult or failed airway.

Non-depolarizing versus Depolarizing Agent for Rapid Sequence Intubation

Succinylcholine is still the most commonly used NMB in prehospital RSI, and is the drug of choice for RSI in the ED and anesthesia. Of the ND-NMBs, rocuronium (0.6-1.2 mg/kg dose) is the most commonly used paralytic agents for RSI because of its rapid onset and short duration with vecuronium (0.15 mg/kg/dose) as a second choice. Succinylcholine's advantages include rapid onset and offset (ie, short duration of action), profound depth of neuromuscular blockade, and better intubating conditions. Comparative trials of succinylcholine with rocuronium found that succinylcholine (1 mg/kg) resulted in superior intubation conditions when compared with rocuronium (0.6 mg/kg). However, a low dose of rocuronium was used. Another recent study also noted similar results with succinylcholine (1 mg/kg) providing superior intubation conditions when compared with rocuronium (again, a lower dose 0.6 mg/kg was used) with no difference in the incidence of adverse airway effects.

Use of Non-depolarizing Neuromuscular Blocking Agents as Pretreatment

The ND-NMBs in a dose that is approximately 10% of the intubating dose can be used as a pretreatment for succinylcholine to prevent fasciculation's and their side effects. Rocuronium is the most commonly used ND-NMB because of its rapid onset, and it can be given 1.5 to 3 minutes before the induction of anesthesia. In clinical practice, the ND-NMB is generally administered 2 minutes before giving the intubating dose of succinylcholine. Although defasciculation is achieved, there are several confounding issues to consider. Giving ND-NMB increases the muscle's resistance to succinylcholine's action such that increasing the succinylcholine dose by 50% is recommended. Use of a ND-NMB may result in less favorable conditions for tracheal intubation and slow the onset of succinylcholine. Perhaps, more importantly, for the emergent intubation in the ED is the extra time (about 2 or more minutes) added to the procedure before intubation occurs. Some physicians also use fasciculations as a clue to when neuromuscular blockade has occurred, and conditions are ready for ET tube placement. Use of a defasciculating dose of ND-NMB adds another drug to RSI (with the additional risk of possible side effects/complications and drug errors), another step, and additional time to the process.

Timing or the use of a small subparalyzing dose of a ND-NMB has several problems as well. There is a danger of aspiration, difficulty swallowing, and uncomfortable visual disturbances for the patient with partial neuromuscular block.

A drug familiar to emergency medicine, lidocaine, can be used as an alternative to ND-NMB for priming before succinylcholine administration. Lidocaine is effective in minimizing or preventing the fasciculations with their side effects that occur after succinylcholine administration. The dose is 1.5 mg/kg of lidocaine.

Modification of Rapid Sequence Intubation

"Facilitated intubation" refers to the use of a sedative only (without a paralytic) to pharmacologically assist with intubation. Facilitated intubation, also referred to as "pharmacologically assisted intubation," has been recommended by some physicians in specific circumstances because it does not involve neuromuscular blockade. Some advocate the avoidance of a neuromuscular paralysis and the use of sedation alone ("facilitated intubation") in clinical scenarios in which a difficult airway is anticipated. For facilitated intubation, the most common sedative used has been etomidate, although midazolam has also been used. Proponents of facilitated intubation suggest that there may be clinical scenarios in which paralysis is not an option.

What Went Wrong?

Etomidate as a Sole Agent for Endotracheal Intubation in the Prehospital Air Medical Setting; *Bozeman WP, Young S (University of Florida, Jacksonville, FL; Baptist/St. Vincent's Health Services, Jacksonville, FL)* Air Med J. 2002;21:32-36

Introduction

Advanced airway management techniques, including medications, are routinely used in prehospital settings. In the authors' helicopter transport service, the rapid-onset anesthetic has been used for several years to facilitate endotracheal intubation. They report their experience with etomidate as the sole agent used to promote intubation, without paralytics.

Patients and Findings

The 2-year experience included 50 patients receiving etomidate to facilitate endotracheal intubation during air transport. In 44 of these, etomidate was the sole agent used. The intubation success rate was 89%, with the remaining 11% of intubations being unsuccessful. Sixteen percent of the intubations were considered difficult, requiring three or more attempts or repeated doses of etomidate. The mean etomidate dose was 0.5 mg/kg. Eight patients vomited, but there were no cases of aspiration. Three patients had trismus or clenched jaws, which precluded successful intubation. One child had seizure-like activity after intubation.

Conclusion

Etomidate may be used on its own to facilitate endotracheal intubation in the field. However, this approach is recommended only when rapid sequence intubation techniques with paralysis are contraindicated or undesirable.

Summary

RSI is the process involving administration of a sedative (ie, induction agent) followed almost immediately by an NMB to facilitate endotracheal intubation. The procedure of RSI generally consists of seven steps: preparation, preoxygenation, pretreatment, paralysis with induction, protection and positioning, placement of the endotracheal tube, and postintubation management. The purpose of RSI is to make emergent intubation easier and safer, thereby increasing the success rate of intubation while decreasing the complications. Possible disadvantages are complications from the additional drugs, prolonged intubation with hypoxia, and precipitating an emergent or crash airway. Controversy has arisen regarding various steps in RSI; however, RSI remains the standard of care in emergency medicine airway management.

REVIEW QUESTIONS

1. **All of the following are indications for rapid sequence intubation utilizing succinylcholine except:**
   A. trauma patients with Glasgow Coma Scale of 9 or less with gag reflex.
   B. trauma patients with significant facial trauma and poor airway control.
   C. closed head injury or major stroke with unconsciousness.
   D. burn patients with airway involvement and inevitable airway loss.
   E. respiratory exhaustion such as severe asthma, CHF or COPD with hypoxia.
   F. overdoses with altered mental status where loss of airway is inevitable.
   G. history of malignant hyperthermia.

   Correct answer is g.

2. **The adult dosage of succinylcholine is:**
   A. 1.5 mg/kg.
   B. 2.5 mg/kg.
   C. 0.5 mg/kg.
   D. 0.75 mg/kg.

Correct answer is a.

3. **The adult dosage of etomidate is:**
   A. 0.1 mg/kg.
   B. 0.3 mg/kg.
   C. 0.5 mg/kg.
   D. 0.6 mg/kg.

Correct answer is b.

4. **The adult dosage for ketamine is:**
   A. 1-2 mg/kg.
   B. 3-5 mg/kg.
   C. 0.3 mg/kg.
   D. 0.1-0.2 mg/kg.

Correct answer is a.

5. **The adult dosage for fentanyl is:**
   A. 1-2 µg/kg.
   B. 3-5 µg/kg.
   C. 0.3 µg/kg.
   D. 0.1-0.2 µg/kg.

Correct answer is a.

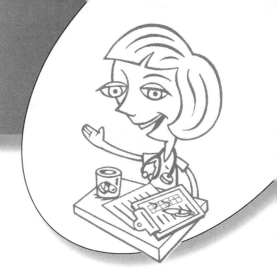

chapter **9**

Endotracheal Intubation

At the end of this chapter, you will be able to:

1. Know the indications for endotracheal intubation.

2. Prepare for and perform safe endotracheal intubation.

3. Identify the patient who is likely to be a "difficult intubation."

4. Have a methodical approach to the management of a "difficult intubation."

5. Know and be able to perform the range of available options in the management of the "difficult intubation."

KEY TERMS

Backward, Upward, Rightward, Pressure (BURP)
Esophageal intubation
Head tilt
Jaw thrust
Macintosh blade
Nasopharyngeal airway
Oropharyngeal airway
Vagal stimulation

Scenario

Your paramedic unit has been dispatched to a difficulty breathing call. The patient's husband has called for his wife who is having dyspnea. Upon arrival you find a 76-year-old woman who is conscious and is in obvious respiratory distress. The patient's husband describes a worsening of swelling in her legs since she stopped taking her water pills. He states she stopped taking the pills because of leg cramps. He states she also takes a heart pill daily. The patient complains of a persistent nonproductive cough that is worse if she lies down. When you ask her what her primary complaint is, she anxiously says, "I.... Can't...Breathe." Her pulse is 110 and irregular, respirations are 28 shallow and labored, and her BP is 190/100. There are wet rales over both lung bases. She has 3+ pitting edema of the lower legs. Pulse oximeter reading is 85%. You are 30 minutes from the hospital.

What is your treatment for this patient?

Introduction

The sharp contrast between the elective patient in an operating room (OR) and the critically ill patient requiring endotracheal intubation in the remote prehospital venue is vast and certainly can become problematic. The elective ambulatory surgical patient characteristically, has received nothing by mouth (NPO) for more than 6 to 8 hours, and has undergone a history and physical examination with appropriate preoperative screening tests. In contrast, in an "emergency" when a paramedic must intubate, an abridged history and physical examination contributes further to compromised patient safety. This chapter focuses on the immediate airway-related consequences that could be considered significant and potentially life-threatening. Although important, dental damage awareness, lip and oral cavity lacerations will not be discussed in this chapter. The consequence of most airway-related complications involves hypoxemia. Complications such as esophageal intubation (EI), regurgitation, aspiration, multiple intubation attempts, and main stem bronchus intubation (MSBI) may each, singly or in combination, lead to oxygen (O_2) desaturation. In an attempt to prevent or limit desaturation during the intubation process and provide a margin of safety in the event of airway difficulties, efforts to provide adequate O_2 reserve should be aggressively pursued. Preoxygenation incorporating either 4 to 8 maximal forced vital capacity breaths of 100% O_2 or 4 minutes of 100% O_2 by using a tight-fitting face mask effectively elevates the PaO_2 reliably in the otherwise stable patient. The critically ill patient may be difficult to administer standard noninvasive O_2 therapy. Despite optimal preoxygenation, pulse oximetry oxygen saturation (SpO_2) may barely clear the 90% saturation. This range equals arterial oxygen tensions in the 55 to 100 mm Hg range, rendering the patient at risk for potentially rapid desaturation. Hypoxemia may be exaggerated if multiple intubation attempts, esophageal intubation, aspiration, uncorrected MSBI, or loss of the airway complicates the intervention.

Indications for Endotracheal Intubation

Typically there are *four main* reasons to intubate:

1. Respiratory failure
2. Impending respiratory failure
3. Relief of airway obstruction
4. Airway protection

Specific Criteria for Intubation

Subjective Criteria for Intubation/Ventilation

- Airway obstruction, real or impending (epiglottitis, burn, tumors, etc)
- Aspiration, real or impending (decreased LOC, drug OD, etc)
- Clinical respiratory failure (tachypnea, tachycardia, cyanosis, diaphoresis, decreased LOC, pulsus paradoxus)
- Tracheal bronchial toilet (unable to clear secretions; COPD with pneumonia)
- Shock not responsive to medical management within 30 minutes (respiratory muscles may use up to 25% of cardiac output; septic shock is a good example)

Objective Criteria for Intubation/Ventilation (Less Important Than Clinical Criteria)

- Oxygenation (PaO_2 measures oxygenation) $PaO_2 < 70$ mm Hg with FIO_2 at least 70%.
- A-a gradient > 350 mm Hg (normal 15, up to 37 with age)
- Ventilation (PCO_2 measures ventilation)
  - $PaCO_2 > 60$ mm Hg in normal adults (not COPD)
  - RR > 35 per minutes in adults
  - $PaCO_2 > 35$ mm Hg in status asthmaticus
  - pH < 7.20 in COPD

Mechanics
Vital capacity < 15 mL/kg (normal is 70 mL/kg)

Complications of Endotracheal Intubation

1. Vomiting and aspiration
2. Hypoxemia with resulting dysrhythmias and/or hypotension
3. Esophageal intubation
4. Chipped or dislodged teeth
5. Trauma to upper airway, tracheal mucosa, or vocal cords
6. Vagal nerve stimulation with secondary bradycardia or hypotension
7. Laryngospasm
8. Failure to intubate

Adverse Complications and Interventions to Endotracheal Intubation

1. **Vomiting:** Stop intubation attempt, suction oropharynx, and ventilate with 100% O_2.
2. **Hypoxemia:** Stop intubation attempt and ventilate with 100% O_2. Emergency drugs will be administered by the paramedic when needed for control of dysrhythmias.
3. **Esophageal intubation:** Remove the endotracheal (ET) tube and ventilate with 100% O_2. Reattempt tracheal intubation when the patient is well oxygenated (Table 9-1).

TABLE 9-1 Complications of Endotracheal Intubation

Complication	Prevention	Management
Missing or broken teeth	Remove teeth prior; avoid using upper teeth as a fulcrum for the laryngoscope blade.	In-hospital a chest x-ray to rule out aspiration.
Clenched teeth		Paralytic medication
Air leak	Check cuff prior to intubation	Inject more air or change tube using a guide wire.
Inability to visualize the cords	Proper patient positioning, proper laryngoscope blade size, and proper suction.	Reposition, choose a different blade, adequate suction.
Esophageal intubation	Visualize the cords.	Remove tube, reoxygenate and reinsert.
Right lung intubation	Avoid excessive tube advancement.	Deflate cuff, re-position and re-inflate.
Laryngospasm	Spray vocal cords with 2% lidocaine.	Benzodiazepine or paralytic medication.
Failure to intubate	None	Have an alternative plan prepared, ie, BVM, supraglottic airway, cricothyroidotomy.

4. **Chipped or dislodged teeth:** Remove these from the airway to prevent their aspiration.

5. **Trauma to the airway mucosa or vocal cords:** Take steps to minimize further damage. Suction the airway of blood if necessary to maintain visualization of anatomical structures.

6. **Vagal stimulation:** Stop intubation attempt and ventilate with 100% O_2. Emergency drugs will be administered by the paramedic when necessary.

7. **Laryngospasm:** Stop intubation attempt and ventilate with 100% O_2. Anesthetize the airway as needed prior to another attempt at intubation; neuromuscular blockade may be necessary.

8. **Failure to intubate:** The necessary steps for emergent cricothyrotomy or tracheostomy must be performed. The paramedic will perform one of these procedures, or he/she will contact personnel who are expert in the performing these techniques. Assistance should be provided as requested and needed throughout the procedure.

Equipment and Materials

- ETs of the estimated size needed, one-half size larger, and one-half size smaller (Figure 9-1):
  - the formula for estimating tube size in pediatric patients up to age 12 is (age in years + 16)/4.
  - adult male 7.5 to 9.0 (8.0) and should be 21 to 24 cm at the lip line
  - adult female 7.0 to 8.5 (7.0) and should be at 18 to 22 cm at the lip line
- Bag-valve-mask and appropriate sized mask
- Tonsil tip suction (Yankauer)
- Laryngoscope and blades with functional bulbs
- Stylet
- 20 cc syringe
- ET fixation device (commercial tube holder) or tape
- Oral airways
- Pulse oximeter
- Cardiac monitor
- $EtCO_2$ mainstream module with cable and adapter
- Cervical collar

Anatomy of an Endotracheal Tube

Assessment

Airway control is paramount in any prehospital setting. It must always be assessed first, and if any compromise or potential compromise is found, this must be dealt with as a first priority.

An airway must be:

1. **Patent:** Having a patent airway is an absolute first priority for any patient. An obstructed airway can be actual (ie, partially or completely obstructed) or potential (ie, airway burns which may result in progressive obstruction over the following few hours).

2. **Protected:** This is a relative priority. It does not take priority over the initial assessment and management of a patient's breathing and circulation. An airway is unprotected when the normal protective reflexes are absent. This is most commonly associated with a decreased level of consciousness. A Glasgow Coma Scale (GCS) of 8 or less is usually associated with an

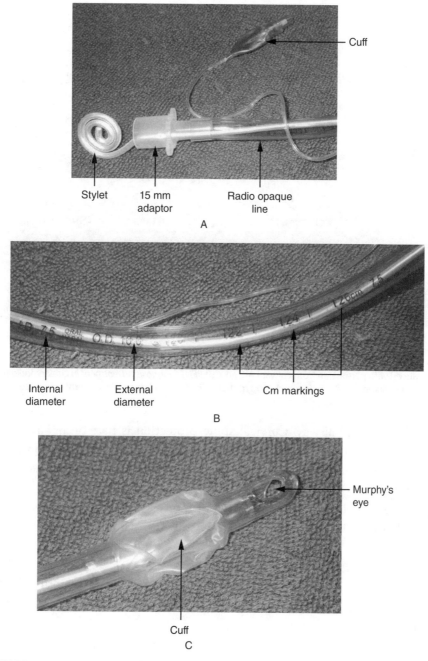

FIGURE 9-1 • (A, B, C) Endotracheal tube, photo by Peter A. DiPrima Jr.

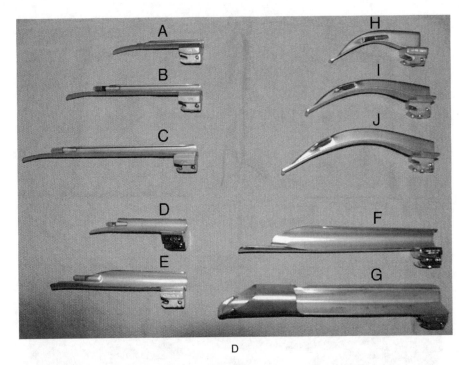

D

FIGURE 9-1D • Anatomy of the laryngoscope blade.
Reproduced with permission from Lalwani AK, ed. *CURRENT Diagnosis & Treatment in Otolaryngology—Head & Neck Surgery*. 3rd ed. New York: Copyright © McGraw-Hill Education. All rights reserved.

unprotected airway. Cervical spine protection is part of airway assessment and management. Any patient with a decreased level of consciousness, who has had trauma to the head or neck, or complains of neck pain, should be treated as having a potential cervical spine injury until proved otherwise. In-line immobilization of the cervical spine or protection by a hard cervical collar must be provided while manipulating the airway.

Airway Assessment
Assessment usually involves examination before history as the majority of cases of airway compromise, either actual or potential, are evident by simple observation.

Examination—Looking for:

- Signs of complete obstruction
  - no air movement present
  - grabbing at throat

- paradoxical breathing with extreme respiratory distress (ie, abdomen moves inward while chest expands during attempted inspiration)
  - cyanosis
  - agitation
- Signs of partial obstruction
  - Still some air movement present
  - Stridor, cough, self-posturing if patient is conscious (ie, sitting up and leaning forward)
  - Use of accessory muscles
  - Cyanosis while breathing room air is a late sign of partial upper airway obstruction
- Signs of potential obstruction
  - Normal air movement
  - None of the above features relating to partial obstruction
  - Swollen face, swollen tongue, sore throat, external neck trauma, circumferential neck burns, sooty sputum, burnt mouth/tongue/nasal hairs, history of fire or explosion in an enclosed space
- Signs suggestive of difficult intubation
  - Signs of a nonprotected airway
  - GCS of 8 or less
  - Absent gag/cough reflex

History

- Symptoms of partial airway obstruction
- Voice changes, cough, sore throat
- Features which suggest potential airway obstruction
  - burns in an enclosed space
  - history of difficult intubation

Simple Airway Opening Maneuvers

- **Head tilt:** This maneuver is performed behind or beside the patient's head, placing the head in the sniffing position (ie, with the neck flexed and the head extended. This is contraindicated in cases of potential or actual cervical spine injury). Great care must be taken in small children to avoid hyperextension of the head as this may occlude the airway.

- **Chin lift:** This is performed from behind or beside the patient's head. Grip the chin from behind by placing your thumb below the lower lip, slightly retracting it, and your fingers on the underside of the chin. With this "pistol grip" pull the mandible forward and upward. This lifts the tongue away from the posterior wall of the pharynx.

- **Jaw thrust:** This is performed from a position behind the patient's head. Place your hands on either side of the head with the little fingers behind the angles of the mandible. Then lift the mandible forward, which lifts the tongue away from the posterior wall of the pharynx. This is the method of choice in patients with cervical spine injury.

Simple Artificial Airway Openers

Oropharyngeal Airway
This is easy to insert. The correct size is that where the length from the flange to posterior tip reaches from the incisors to the angle of the mandible. An average adult will take a size 3. In adults it is inserted into the mouth upside down and then rotated through 180 degrees on reaching the oropharynx. In children it is inserted in the position of function (a tongue depressor may be used to hold the tongue clear) as the rotation may injure the soft palate.

Advantages
- Cheap
- Easy
- Safe and effective

Disadvantages
- Does not protect the airway
- If the patient is conscious there may be gagging, coughing, straining, and vomiting.

Complications
- Failed placement causing airway obstruction
- Trauma
- Vomiting and aspiration

Nasopharyngeal Airway

This is a softer artificial airway than the oropharyngeal and it is passed along the floor of the nose into the pharynx. The correct size is that with a length from flange to tip adequate to reach from the nares to the angle of the mandible. It must be lubricated prior to insertion.

Advantages

- Can be used in patient with clenched jaw
- Does not cause as much gagging as an oropharyngeal airway
- Does not have to negotiate the tongue

Disadvantages

- More difficult to insert
- Cannot use if possible fracture to base of skull, facial fractures
- Does not protect the airway
- Hemorrhage more likely

Complications

- As for oropharyngeal airway with the addition of intracranial placement in the setting of fractured base of skull.

None of these simple airway opening techniques/devices will provide airway protection.

Airway Suction

Obstruction of the airway may occur due to pooling of secretions, blood, vomit, or other debris in the airway. Suctioning of the airway should be done with an appropriate size sucker and in conjunction with airway opening maneuvers.

1. Ensure that suction tubing is attached to the suction outlet, via a suction bottle for collection of secretions/vomitus.
2. Tubing should be large bore to facilitate passage of blood or vomitus.
3. The catheter should be rigid, with a rigid tip and large bore openings.
4. In conjunction with basic airway opening techniques the suction catheter should be gently inserted into the pharynx and mouth, and secretions removed. It may be necessary to clear the tip to remove large particulate matter.
5. The placing of an oropharyngeal airway will prevent the patient from biting down on the suction catheter.

Endotracheal Intubation Procedure

Preparing the Patient

1. Secure IV access and flush cannula to ensure patency.

2. If the need for intubation is not immediate, treat or exclude comorbid conditions which may be exacerbated by intubation (ie, pneumothorax, hypovolemia).

3. Position the patient supine with the head extended and the neck flexed. This may be facilitated by a thin pillow being placed under the head. This position will not only maintain an open airway to aid bag-valve ventilation, but will also aid intubation (Figure 9-2).

4. Cervical spine precautions should be observed where there is a likelihood of cervical spine injury. (Use in line stabilization.)

5. Preoxygenate with 100% O_2 for 5 minutes. This is usually achieved using a bag-valve mask attached to O_2. If the patient is breathing spontaneously manual ventilation is not necessary and may risk gastric distension and regurgitation/aspiration.

6. Initiate cardiac monitoring, pulse oximetry and $EtCO_2$ monitoring.

Intubation Procedure

1. Gather and prepare/test equipment.

2. Connect the manual resuscitator and mask to O_2.

3. Test the pilot balloon on the ET, insert the stylet, and lubricate the tube with water-soluble jelly.

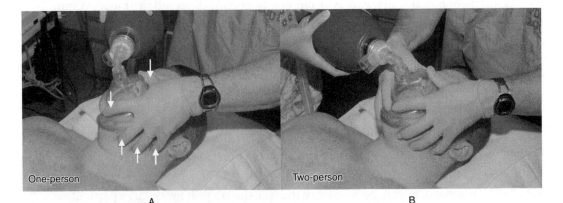

One-person

Two-person

A

B

FIGURE 9-2 • (A and B) Bag-valve mask ventilation.
Reproduced with permission from Knoop KJ, Stack LB, Storrow AB, Thurman RJ, eds. *The Atlas of Emergency Medicine.* 3rd ed. New York: Copyright © McGraw-Hill Education. All rights reserved.

4. Test and tighten the laryngoscope blades' bulbs.

5. Don the appropriate universal precautions apparel.

6. Position the patient appropriately.

7. Hyperoxygenate the patient with resuscitation bag, mask, and 100% O_2.

8. Have someone to assist the paramedic as needed during the intubation. (With suctioning, patient repositioning, supplies, cricoid pressure, and bag-valve mask ventilation.)

   To maximize the potential exposure of the glottic opening, it is essential that the oral axis, the pharyngeal axis, and the laryngeal axis approximate a straight line thereby affording the shortest distance from the teeth to the glottic opening (Figure 9-3). This is best accomplished by placing the supine patient in the position described as the "sniffing" position. Elevating (using a blanket, folded towel, foam rest, etc) the occiput approximately 10 cm higher than the shoulder blades provides the necessary cervical flexion to better align the laryngeal and pharyngeal axes. Extension of the head on the atlanto-occipital joint by the paramedic's freehand (or by an assistant) will serve to maximally align the oral axis with the laryngeal and pharyngeal axes. A significant number of difficult or failed intubations have been attributed to poor positioning.

9. Monitor the O_2 saturation using the pulse oximeter and if saturation falls below 90% perform re-oxygenation.

10. Place the endotracheal blade into the oropharynx (Figure 9-4).

11. Visualize the opening of the glottis (Figure 9-5).

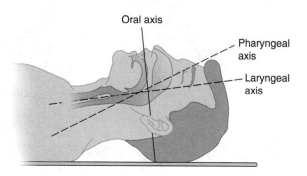

FIGURE 9-3 • Head placement.
Reproduced with permission from Tintinalli JE, Stapczynski JS, Cline DM, Ma OJ, Cydulka RK, Meckler GD, eds. *Tintinalli's Emergency Medicine: A Comprehensive Study Guide*. 7th ed. 2011. New York: Copyright © McGraw-Hill Education. All rights reserved.

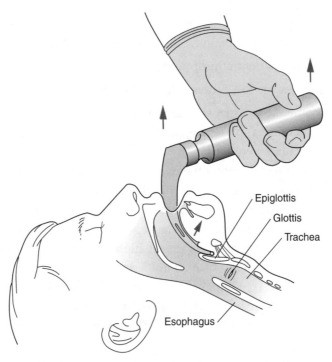

FIGURE 9-4 • Macintosh blade insertion.
Reproduced with permission from Gomella LG, Haist SA, eds. *Clinician's Pocket Reference: The Scut Monkey.* 11th ed. 2007. New York: Copyright © McGraw-Hill Education. All rights reserved.

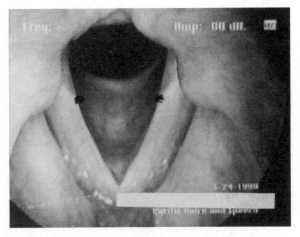

FIGURE 9-5 • Vocal cord visualization.
Reproduced with permission from Lalwani AK, ed. *CURRENT Diagnosis & Treatment in Otolaryngology—Head & Neck Surgery.* 3rd ed. 2012. New York: Copyright © McGraw-Hill Education. All rights reserved. Figure 29-1A.

12. Once the ET is inserted, place $EtCO_2$ adapter between the endotracheal tube and the resuscitation bag.

13. Assure proper placement of the ET by observation of chest expansion and auscultation with manual breaths and presence of adequate $EtCO_2$ waveform (Figure 9-6).

14. After good placement has been confirmed, note the "cm" marking on the tube at the position of the lip or teeth, and secure the tube. The "cm" marking at the lip or teeth should be documented, and monitored to help ascertain whether the tube has shifted in position.

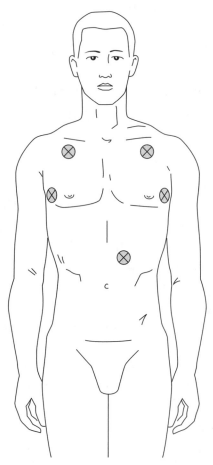

FIGURE 9-6 • Auscultation sites.
Reproduced with permission from Morgan, Jr. GE, Mikhail MS, Murray MJ, eds. *Clinical Anesthesiology.* 4th ed. 2006. New York: Copyright © McGraw-Hill Education. All rights reserved.

15. Document good position of the ET.

16. Continuous $EtCO_2$ monitoring should be performed to assure patency of the airway.

17. Apply a cervical collar to reduce hyperextension and hyperflexion.

Management of the Difficult Endotracheal Intubation

While the patient is being prepared for intubation, if the vocal cords are not observed during laryngoscopy, different maneuvers can be tried to help visualize the glottis. The following steps may provide adequate exposure for direct visualization of the true vocal cords:

1. **Backward, upward, rightward pressure (BURP)**: This applies to a technique to aid visualization of the larynx when the larynx lies caudal and anterior. It refers to the application:

   - **Backward:** to push the larynx backward
   - **Upward:** to push the larynx as superiorly as possible
   - **Rightward:** no more than 2 cm
   - **Pressure:** to the thyroid cartilage (NOT the cricoid)

2. **Use a larger blade**

   In patients with a large lower jaw or deep pharynx, use of a larger, size 4 Macintosh blade (Figure 9-4) rather than the more common size 3 (for consistency) can facilitate the tip of the blade reaching the vallecula for optimal elevation of the epiglottis. Alternatively, using a straight blade such as a Miller 2 or 3 may facilitate intubation.

3. **The lighted stylet**

   A malleable metal or plastic rod with a fiberoptic light source that is passed through the ET to adjust its curvature helps facilitate blind intubation (ie, when the glottis is poorly visualized or not observed). Greater intensity of light visible through the soft tissue of the anterior neck as the light passes beyond the vocal cords helps distinguish the tracheal lumen from the esophagus.

4. **Gum elastic bougie**

   This is an extension of the concept of the introducer. A long piece of elastic material which is semirigid can be directed into the trachea when it is impossible to achieve direct intubation because of an inability to see

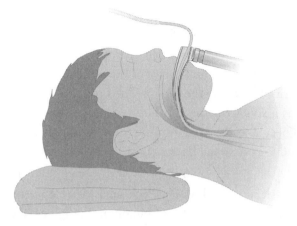

FIGURE 9-7 • Elastic bougie.
Reproduced with permission from Tintinalli JE, Stapczynski JS, Cline DM, Ma OJ, Cydulka RK, Meckler GD, eds. *Tintinalli's Emergency Medicine: A Comprehensive Study Guide*. 7th ed. 2011. New York: Copyright © McGraw-Hill Education. All rights reserved. Figure 30-4.

the cords or because of difficulty in directing the ET between the cords (see Figure 9-7).

Technique

1. Under direct vision using the laryngoscope the bougie is passed between the cords as to where the cords are estimated to be.
2. An appropriate sized ET is then passed over the bougie and into the trachea using the bougie to guide the tube
3. If the tube appears to catch at the cords its advancement may be facilitated by twisting the tube through 180 degrees.
4. The bougie is then removed, leaving the tube in place.

Complications
- Failed intubation
- Trauma to the airway
- Esophageal intubation

Advantages
- Technically simple
- Avoids surgical procedures

Disadvantages

Can be awkward, particularly if ET gets snagged at the cords

- **Fiberoptic intubation:** Pass a flexible fiberoptic bronchoscope through the ET and then through the oral cavity of the patient. Pull the mandible and tongue anterior to expose the larynx. The bronchoscope serves as a visual guide and as a stylet for the ET. The technique may also be used if the patient has been anesthetized; however, loss of muscle tone will allow the epiglottis and tongue to fall back against the posterior pharynx. Pulling the jaw forward is likely to be required.

- **Laryngeal mask airway (LMA):** Place an LMA (ie, a small latex mask mounted on a hollow plastic tube) blindly in the lower pharynx overlying the glottis. The inflatable cuff on the mask wedges the mask in the hypopharynx and helps seal the gastrointestinal tract from the airway (Figure 9-8).

- **Esophageal-tracheal double-lumen airway:** Use a Combitube®, a combined esophageal obturator and tracheal tube (Figure 9-9). This twin-lumen device is inserted without the need for visualization into the oropharynx and usually into the esophagus. It has a low-volume inflatable

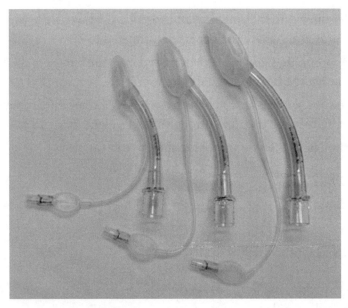

FIGURE 9-8 • Laryngeal mask airway.
Reproduced with permission from Tintinalli JE, Stapczynski JS, Cline DM, Ma OJ, Cydulka RK, Meckler GD, eds. *Tintinalli's Emergency Medicine: A Comprehensive Study Guide.* 7th ed. 2011. New York: Copyright © McGraw-Hill Education. All rights reserved.

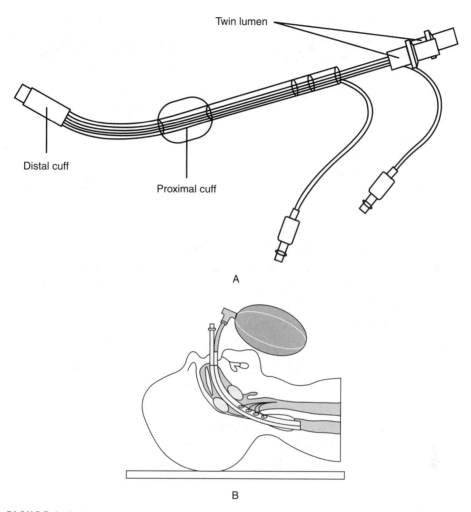

FIGURE 9-9 • Combitube.
Reproduced with permission from Lalwani AK, ed. *CURRENT Diagnosis & Treatment in Otolaryngology—Head & Neck Surgery*. 3rd ed. 2012. New York: Copyright © McGraw-Hill Education. All rights reserved

distal cuff and a much larger proximal cuff designed to occlude the oro and nasopharynx. If the tube has entered the trachea, ventilation is achieved through the distal lumen as with a standard ET. More commonly, the device enters the esophagus and ventilation is achieved through multiple openings in the tube situated above the distal cuff. In the latter case, the proximal and distal cuffs must be inflated to prevent air from escaping through the esophagus or back out of the oropharynx and nasopharynx.

TABLE 9-2 Diseases and Syndromes That Are Likely to Render Bag-Valve Mask Ventilation and Endotracheal Intubation Difficult	
Acromegaly	Ankylosing spondylitis
Stylohyoid ligament calcification	Fetal alcohol syndrome
Cervical osteoarthritis	Cockayne's syndrome
Pierre Robin syndrome	Rheumatoid arthritis
Temporomandibular joint dysfunction	Still's disease
Treacher Collins syndrome	Tracheal agenesis

- **Retrograde guide wire:** A Seldinger guide wire is inserted by needle through the cricothyroid membrane and bounced toward the mouth off the back wall of the trachea. It is then retrieved in the mouth. The ET is introduced through the vocal cords over the guide wire, which is removed as the tube passes down the trachea.

In the emergency setting, there may be little time to perform an adequate assessment of the airway. Patients may be unconscious, in respiratory distress, or cyanotic. Injuries may limit or preclude the establishment of a mask airway (see Table 9-2). In these settings, the individual most experienced in tracheal intubation should perform direct laryngoscopy to evaluate the airway and attempt the intubation. Even in the case of cervical injury, where in-line traction for stabilization of the neck must be performed by an assistant, the technique of direct laryngoscopy is most likely the quickest method to secure the airway. However, even in the most urgent of clinical situations, back-up plans, including the use of a fiber optic camera and the process of establishing a surgical airway, must be considered.

The patient with a full stomach presents special challenges in securing an airway. Here the risk of aspiration of stomach contents is weighed against the urgency of establishing an artificial airway. While RSI may be a viable solution in the patient with a known history of easy mask ventilation and a class I view (Mallampati) of the vocal cords, the approach to the unknown patient with a receding chin, protruding incisors, and a small mouth opening will be quite different (Figure 9-10).

Here the possibility of an awake intubation must be considered. In the most-dire of circumstances, the issue of treating aspiration versus hypoxic neurological damage must play a role in the decision-making process.

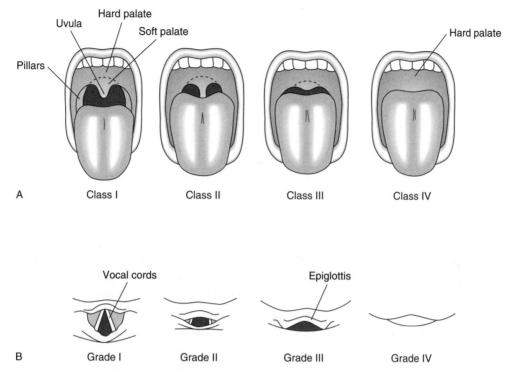

FIGURE 9-10 • A and B Mallampati score.
From Mallampati SR: Clinical signs to predict difficult tracheal intubation [hypothesis].
Can Anaesth Soc J. 1983;30:316, with kind permission from Springer+Business Media B.V.

Intoxicated patients are considered to have a full stomach. These patients may also be uncooperative and/or combative. This may be as a result of injury, intoxication, or hypoxemia. Such patients may require sedation prior to airway evaluation. Use of sedation must be approached with caution in consideration of the possibility of respiratory compromise. Oversedation is an easy, lethal complication. Injury to the chest and thorax may limit the positioning of the patient and may compromise the mechanics of oxygenation and ventilation. Consideration must be given to the possibility of trauma to the tracheobronchial tree. A pneumothorax or an injury to a main-stem bronchus may require a different approach to airway management, including the use of different airway devices. Injuries to the head and neck, including facial burns and maxillofacial injuries, may severely limit the ability to examine the upper airway. Damage to facial structures may compromise the mask fit and cause swelling that may impinge on the upper airway. Injuries to the eye often limit access to the nose and mouth region. Additionally, injuries to the globe may necessitate avoidance of increased intracranial pressure that may often accompany laryngoscopy and intubation. In patients with suspected injuries of the neck and/or cervical spine, special precautions must be utilized to ensure that management of the airway causes no further damage.

Summary

The difficult airway, although relatively rare, still occurs with a frequency sufficient to require that all personnel associated with airway management be familiar with methods to use when confronted with a challenging airway. The most effective means of anticipating a difficult airway lies in an integrated approach utilizing the history, physical examination, and the patient's current medical condition. The most effective manner of dealing with a difficult airway involves proper anticipation, patient preparation, and the development of practical, well thought out contingency plans.

Orotracheal intubation is both common and lifesaving. It is the primary and preferred method of airway management. Every paramedic must master the skill. With proper preparation, definitive control of the airway can be obtained. This assures that patients can be oxygenated and ventilated when they cannot do this on their own. Good team leadership skills are nearly as important as physical dexterity, and assure an orderly and quick procedure. Rapid patient assessment is important to prevent complications. As stated earlier, if endotracheal intubation is unsuccessful, another form of intubation, insertion of a supraglottic airway or a surgical airway should be performed.

REVIEW QUESTIONS

1. **Complications of endotracheal intubation:**
   A. Vomiting and aspiration.
   B. Hypoxemia with resulting dysrhythmias and/or hypotension.
   C. Esophageal intubation.
   D. Chipped or dislodged teeth.
   E. All the above are correct.

   Correct answer is e.

2. **Indications for endotracheal intubation include respiratory failure, impending respiratory failure, relief of airway obstruction, and airway protection.**

   A. True.
   B. False.

Correct answer is a.

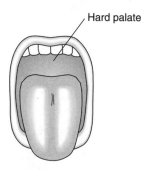

Hard palate

From Mallampati SR: Clinical signs to predict difficult tracheal intubation [hypothesis]. *Can Anaesth Soc J.* 1983;30:316, with kind permission from Springer+Business Media B.V.

3. **Figure 9-11 depicts what Mallampati score?**

   A. Class I.
   B. Class II.
   C. Class III.
   D. Class IV.

Correct answer is d.

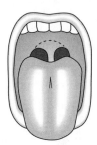

From Mallampati SR: Clinical signs to predict difficult tracheal intubation [hypothesis]. *Can Anaesth Soc J.* 1983;30:316, with kind permission from Springer+Business Media B.V.

4. **Figure 9-12 depicts what Mallampati Score?**

   A. Class I.
   B. Class II.
   C. Class III.
   D. Class IV.

Correct answer is b.

5. **The *BURP* maneuver stands for:**

   A. backward, upward, leftward pressure.

   B. backward, upward, rightward pressure.

   C. Both a and b are correct.

   D. None of the above are correct.

Correct answer is b.

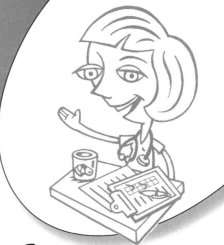

chapter **10**

Airway Devices for Difficult Airway Management, Supraglottic Airway Devices

LEARNING OBJECTIVES

At the end of this chapter, you will be able to:

1. Describe selection of a supraglottic airway device to perform ventilation.
2. List the equipment used to perform insertion of the supraglottic airway.
3. Record the steps to insert a supraglottic airway.
4. Describe complications of insertion of a supraglottic airway.
5. Explain extubation of a supraglottic airway.
6. Identify the indications for extubation of a supraglottic airway.
7. Describe the complications of extubation of a supraglottic airway.

KEY TERMS

Esophageal-tracheal combitube
Laryngeal mask airway (LMA)
Supraglottic airway devices (SAD)

Scenario

A basic life support crew is on scene at local housing project and are treating an obese man with a poly drug overdose; nortryptilline, diazepam, venlafaxine, and trazadone. They are requesting paramedics. As you arrive on scene the emergency medical technician (EMT) tells you that the patient is obtunded and has a low BP of 100/60. They have the patient totally flat on the gurney, they are ventilating him but can't get effective air movement, the patient's nose and fingers are somewhere between purple and black in color. "Respiratory collapse!" the EMT shouts, "I can't bag him!" The patient looks to be about 5'7" and you estimate a weight of about 400 lbs. His neck is short to the point of being non-existent.

What do you do now?

The crash difficult airway is not an uncommon scenario in emergency medical services (EMS). This presents us with the absolute worst airway situation; the patient is hypoxic and near death, the airway is difficult to manage and we have had no time to prepare for a nuanced attempt at airway management. We all know by looking at this patient with a BMI above 40 and no neck that the airway is going to be a challenge.

Introduction

Supraglottic airway devices (SAD) play an important role in the management of patients with difficult airways. Unlike other alternatives to standard endotracheal intubation, (ie, videolaryngoscopy or intubation stylets) they enable ventilation even in patients with difficult facemask ventilation and simultaneous use as a conduit for tracheal intubation. Insertion is usually atraumatic, their use is familiar from elective anesthesia, and compared with tracheal intubation is easier to learn for users with limited experienced in airway management. Use of SADs during difficult airway management is widely recommended in many guidelines for the operating room and in the prehospital setting. As paramedics we spend a respectable part of our career training and learning how to properly maintain the airway. Theoretically, every paramedic should be familiar with, and well-practiced in a variety of the airway techniques that are available, so that when an airway problem occurs, it can be managed with a solid collection of information and experience. However, with rapid advancements in airway management technology, many of the newer airway devices are foreign to most paramedics. In the past few years, a number of supraglottic airway devices have been introduced in the clinical practice of airway management, trying to offer a simple and effective alternative to the endotracheal intubation.

Supraglottic airway devices are devices that ventilate patients by delivering oxygen above the level of the vocal cords and are designed to overcome the disadvantages of endotracheal intubation such as; soft tissue damage, tooth, vocal cords, laryngeal and tracheal damage, exaggerated hemodynamic response, and barotrauma. The advantages of the supraglottic airway device include avoidance of laryngoscopy, less invasive for the respiratory tract, better tolerated by patients, increased ease of placement, improved hemodynamic stability in emergent situations, less coughing, less sore throat, hands-free airway, and easier placement by inexperienced personal. The American Society of Anesthesiologists' Task Force on Management of the Difficult Airway, suggests considering the use of the supraglottic airway devices (such as laryngeal mask airway, king, or combitube) when intubation problems occur in patients with a previously unrecognized difficult airway, especially in a "cannot ventilate, cannot intubate" situation.

Laryngeal Mask Airway

The laryngeal mask airway (LMA) has been described as the missing link between the facemask and the tracheal tube and it has gained widespread popularity. The LMA is a supraglottic airway device developed by British anesthesiologist, Dr. Archie Brain. It has been in use since 1988. Initially designed for use in the operating room as a method of elective ventilation, it is a good alternative to bag-valve-mask ventilation, freeing the hands of the provider with the benefit of less gastric distention. Initially used primarily in the operating room setting, the LMA has more recently come into use in the emergency setting as an important accessory device for management of the difficult airway.

The LMA is shaped like a large endotracheal tube on the proximal end that connects to an elliptical mask on the distal end. It is designed to sit in the patient's hypopharynx and cover the supraglottic structures, thereby allowing relative isolation of the trachea (Figure 10-1).

The LMA is a good airway device in many settings, including the operating room, the emergency department, and out-of-hospital care, because it is easy to use and quick to place, even for the inexperienced provider. It has a success rate of nearly 100% in the operating room, although this may be lower in the emergency setting. Its use results in less gastric distention than with bag-valve-mask ventilation, which reduces but does not eliminate the risk of aspiration.

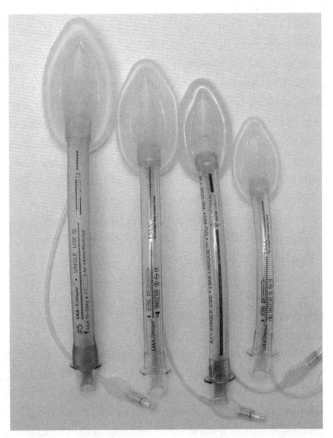

FIGURE 10-1 • LMA.
Reproduced, with permission, from Knoop KJ, Stack LB, Storrow AB, et al. *Atlas of Emergency Medicine.* 3rd ed. 2009. New York: Copyright © McGraw-Hill Education. Fig. 22-46. (Photo contributor: Lawrence B. Stack, MD.)

This may be particularly pertinent in patients who have not fasted before being ventilated.

There are several types of laryngeal mask airways.

The LMA Classic is the original reusable design.

- The LMA Unique is a disposable version, making it ideal for emergency and prehospital settings.

- The LMA Fastrach, an intubating LMA (ILMA), is designed to serve as a conduit for intubation. Although most LMA designs can serve this purpose, the LMA Fastrach has special features that increase the rate of successful intubation and do not limit the size of the endotracheal (ET) tube. These features include an insertion handle, a rigid shaft with anatomical curvature, and an epiglottic elevating bar designed to lift the epiglottis as the ET passes.

- The LMA Flexible has softer tubing. It is not used in the emergency setting.

- The LMA ProSeal has the addition of a channel for the suctioning of gastric contents. It also allows for 50% higher pressures without a leak. However, it does not permit blind intubation and is not currently used in the emergency setting.

- The LMA Supreme, which is a newer design, is similar to the ProSeal and has a built-in bite block.

- Another newer design is the LMA C-Trach, which inserts like the LMA Fastrach and has built-in fiberoptics with a video screen that affords a direct view of the larynx.

Indications

1. **Elective ventilation**

   - The LMA is an acceptable alternative to mask anesthesia in the operating room.

   - It is often used for short procedures when endotracheal intubation is not necessary.

2. **Difficult airway**

   - After failed intubation, the LMA can be used as a rescue device.

   - In the case of the patient who cannot be intubated but can be ventilated, the LMA is a good alternative to continued bag-valve-mask ventilation because LMA is easier to maintain over time and it has been shown to decrease, though not eliminate, aspiration risk.

- In the case of the patient who cannot be intubated or ventilated, a surgical airway is indicated and should not be delayed. However, if the LMA is at hand, it can easily be attempted quickly, while an assistant simultaneously prepares for cricothyroidotomy.

3. **Cardiac arrest**

- The 2010 American Heart Association guidelines indicate the LMA a an acceptable alternative to intubation for airway management in the cardiac arrest patient (Class IIa).
- The LMA may be particularly useful in the prehospital setting, where EMS providers may have less experience with intubation and lower success rates.

4. **Conduit for intubation**

- The LMA can be used as a conduit for intubation, particularly when direct laryngoscopy is unsuccessful.
- An ET tube can be passed directly through the LMA or ILMA. Intubation may also be assisted by a bougie or fiberoptic scope.

5. **Prehospital airway management**

- The LMA is useful in the prehospital setting not only for patients in cardiac arrest but also for managing a difficult airway.
- In patients whom positioning or prolonged extrication does not allow for endotracheal intubation, the LMA can be inserted and allowed for successful airway management until a definitive airway can be established.

6. **Pediatric use**

- Laryngeal mask airways are available in a range of pediatric sizes.

Contraindications

- Absolute contraindications (in all settings, including emergent)
  - cannot open mouth
  - complete upper airway obstruction
- Relative contraindications (in the elective setting)

- increased risk of aspiration
  - prolonged bag-valve-mask ventilation
  - morbid obesity
  - second or third trimester pregnancy
  - patients who have not fasted before ventilation
  - upper gastrointestinal bleed
- suspected or known abnormalities in supraglottic anatomy
- need for high airway pressures (in all but the LMA ProSeal, pressure cannot exceed 20 mm H_2O for effective ventilation.)

Steps in Insertion of the LMA

Step1: Sizing (Table 10-1)

TABLE 10-1 LMA: Recommended Size guidelines	
LMA size	**Patient Weight**
Size 1	Under 5 kg
Size 1.5	5 to 10 kg
Size 2	10 to 20 kg
Size 2.5	20 to 30 kg
Size 3	30 kg to small adult
Size 4	Adult
Size 5	Large adult or poor seal with size 4

Step 2

- Visually inspect the LMA cuff for tears or other abnormalities.
- Inspect the tube to ensure that it is free of blockage or loose particles.
- Deflate the cuff to ensure that it will maintain a vacuum.
- Inflate the cuff to ensure that it does not leak.

Step 3

- Slowly deflate the cuff to form a smooth flat wedge shape which will pass easily around the back of the tongue and behind the epiglottis (Table 10-2).

TABLE 10-2 Maximum Air Inflation	
Cuff	**Maximum Air Inflation**
Size 1	4 mL
Size 1.5	7 mL
Size 2	10 mL
Size 2.5	14 mL
Size 3	20 mL
Size 4	30 mL
Size 5	40 mL

Step 4

- Use a water-soluble lubricant to lubricate the LMA.
- Only lubricate the LMA just prior to insertion.
- Lubricate the back of the mask thoroughly.

Note

- Avoid excessive amounts of lubricanton the anterior surface of the cuff or in the bowl of the mask.
- Inhalation of the lubricant following placement may result in coughing or obstruction.

Step 5

- Extend the head and flex the neck.
- Avoid LMA fold over:
  - assistant pulls the lower jaw downward.
  - visualize the posterior oral airway.
  - ensure that the LMA is not folding over in the oral cavity as it is inserted (Figure 10-2).

Esophageal-Tracheal Combitube

The esophageal-tracheal combitube (ETC) is an easily inserted double lumen-double balloon supraglottic airway device that allows for ventilation independent of its position either in the esophagus or the trachea. Blind insertion results in successful esophageal intubation in nearly all patients. The major indication

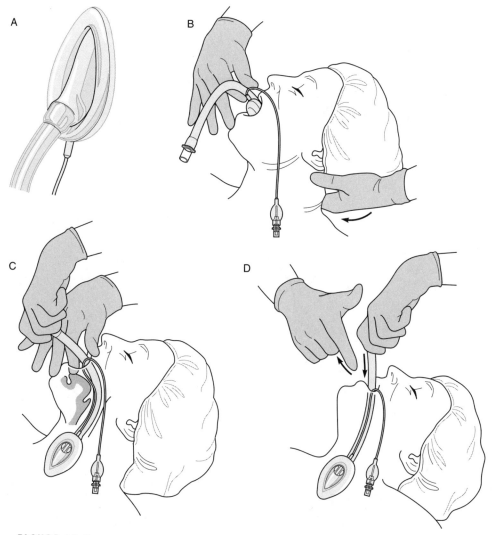

FIGURE 10-2 • LMA Insertion.
Reproduced with permission from LMA North America.

of the ETC is a back-up device for airway management. It is an excellent option for rescue ventilation in both in and out of the hospital environment, as well as in immediate life-threatening cannot ventilate, cannot intubate situations. The advantages of the combitube include rapid airway control without the need for neck or head movement, minimized risk for aspiration, firm fixation of the device after inflation of the oropharyngeal balloon, and it works equally well in either tracheal or esophageal position (Figure 10-3).

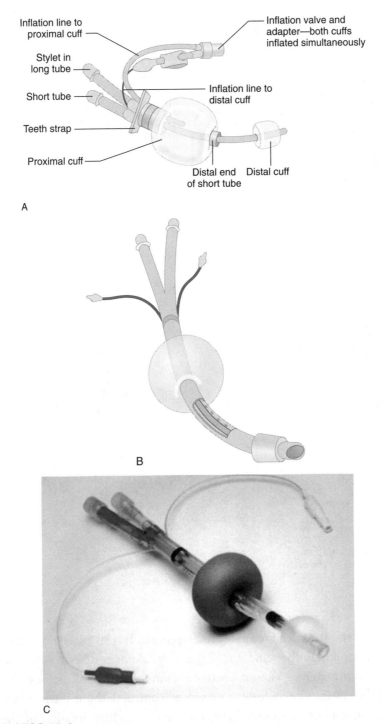

FIGURE 10-3 • Combitube.

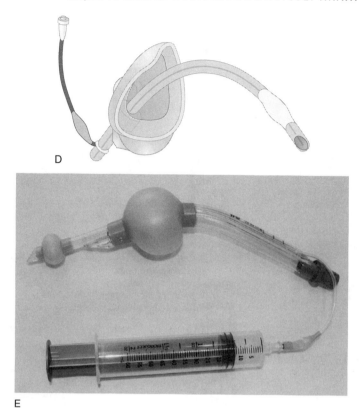

FIGURE 10-3 · *(Continued)*

Laryngeal Tube

The laryngeal tube (LT) is a multiuse, latex-free, single-lumen silicon tube and consists of an airway tube with an approximate angle of 130 degrees, an average diameter of 1.5 mm and two low pressure cuffs (proximal and distal) with two oval apertures placed between them which allows ventilation. The distal balloon (esophageal balloon) seals the airway distally and protects against regurgitation. The proximal balloon (oropharyngeal balloon) seals both the oral and nasal cavity. When the LT is inserted, it lies along the length of the tongue, and the distal tip is positioned in the upper esophagus. During ventilation, air passes into the pharynx and from there over the epiglottis into the trachea, since the mouth, nose, and esophagus are blocked by the balloons. A new single use version of the LT has been recently introduced in the market (Figure 10-4).

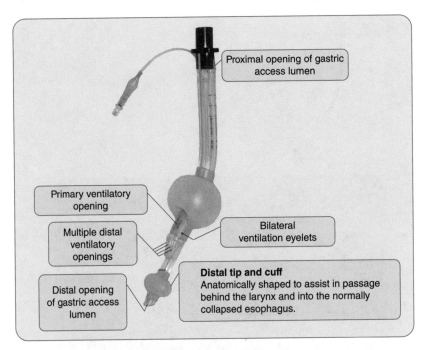

FIGURE 10-4 • Design features exclusive to the King LTS-D.
Reproduced with permission from King LT, King Systems Corporation KLTD EMS In-service Package.

Insertion

1. Apply chin lift and introduce the LT into the corner of the mouth (Figure 10-5).
2. Advance tip under base of tongue, while rotating tube back to midline (Figure 10-6).
3. Without exerting excessive force, advance tube until base of connector is aligned with teeth or gums (Figure 10-7).
4. Inflate cuff according to package reference or volume noted on tube (Figure 10-8).
5. Attach bag valve. While gently bagging, slowly withdraw tube until ventilation is easy and free flowing (large tidal volume with minimal airway pressure) (Figure 10-9).

Contraindications

The LT does not protect the airway from regurgitation and aspiration effects. These contraindications are applicable for routine use of the laryngeal tube:

1. Responsive patients with an intact gag reflex.
2. Patients with known esophageal disease.
3. Patients who have ingested caustic substances.

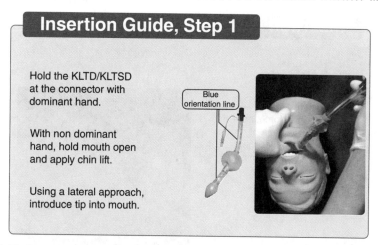

FIGURE 10-5 • Insertion guide, step 1.
Reproduced with permission from King LT, King Systems Corporation KLTD EMS In-service Package.

The newly introduced laryngeal tube suction (LTS) is a further development of the LT which allows better separation of the respiratory and alimentary tracts. The LTS is a latex-free, double lumen silicon tube wherein one lumen is used for ventilation and the other for decompression, suctioning, and gastric tube placement.

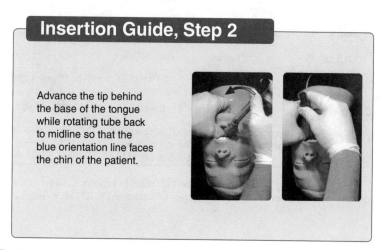

FIGURE 10-6 • Insertion guide, step 2.
Reproduced with permission from King LT, King Systems Corporation KLTD EMS In-service Package.

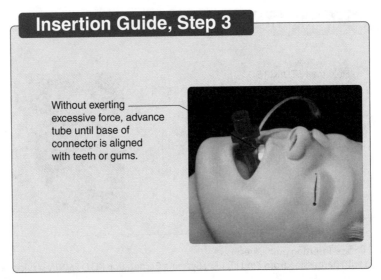

Insertion Guide, Step 3

Without exerting excessive force, advance tube until base of connector is aligned with teeth or gums.

FIGURE 10-7 • Insertion guide, step 3.
Reproduced with permission from King LT, King Systems Corporation KLTD EMS In-service Package.

King LT-D Size	3	4	5
Connector color	Yellow	Red	Purple
Recommended patient height	4–5 ft (122–155 cm)	5–6 ft (155–180 cm)	Greater than 6 ft (180 cm)
Item #	KLTD213	KLTD214	KLTD215
O.D./I.D.	14 mm/10 mm	14 mm/10 mm	14 mm/10 mm
Cuff pressure	60 cm H_2O	60 cm H_2O	60 cm H_2O
Cuff volume	45–60 mL	60–80 mL	70–90 mL

Maximum size fiberoptic bronchoscope: 7.0 mm O.D.,
Maximum size tube exchange catheter: 19 Fr,
Maximum ET tube: 6.0 mm I.D.

FIGURE 10-8 • King LT, King Systems Corporation KLTD EMS In-service Package.
Reproduced with permission from King LT, King Systems Corporation KLTD EMS In-service Package.

Insertion Guide, Step 5

Attach the resuscitator bag to the KLTD/KLTSD.

While bagging the patient, gently withdraw the tube until ventilation becomes easy and free flowing (large tidal volume with minimal airway pressure).

Adjust cuff inflation if necessary to obtain a seal of the airway at the peak ventilatory pressure employed.

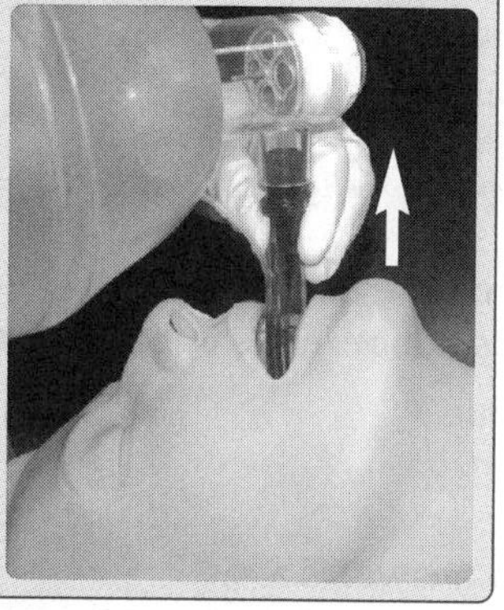

FIGURE 10-9 • Insertion guide, step 5.
Reproduced with permission from King LT, King Systems Corporation KLTD EMS In-service Package.

REVIEW QUESTIONS

1. **Supraglottic airway devices are devices that ventilate patients by delivering oxygen above the level of the vocal cords and are designed to overcome the disadvantages of endotracheal intubation.**

   A. True.
   B. False.

Correct answer is a.

2. **The LT does not protect the airway from regurgitation and aspiration effects. These contraindications are applicable for routine use of the laryngeal tube:**

   A. Responsive patients with an intact gag reflex.
   B. Patients with known esophageal disease.
   C. Patients who have ingested caustic substances.
   D. All of the above are correct.

Correct answer is d.

3. The advantages of the combitube include rapid airway control without the need for neck or head movement, minimized risk for aspiration, firm fixation of the device after inflation of the oropharyngeal balloon, and it works equally well in either tracheal or esophageal position.

   A. True.
   B. False.

Correct answer is a.

4. When the LT is inserted, it lies along the length of the tongue and the distal tip is positioned in the upper esophagus.

   A. True.
   B. False.

Correct answer is a.

5. Regarding the LT, the distal balloon (esophageal balloon) seals the airway distally and protects against regurgitation. The proximal balloon (oropharyngeal balloon) seals both the oral and nasal cavity.

   A. True.
   B. False.

Correct answer is a.

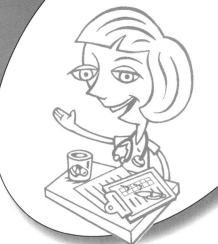

chapter **11**

Special Clinical Considerations for the "Difficult Airway"

LEARNING OBJECTIVES

At the end of this chapter, you will be able to:

1. Describe the unique aspects of pediatric airway management.
2. Review the pediatric airway anatomy and respiratory physiology.
3. Review routine pediatric airway management.
4. Describe how to manage the difficult pediatric airway.

KEY TERMS

Apert syndrome
Bronchiolitis
Bronchopulmonary dysplasia (BPD)
Crackles
Croup
Crouzon syndrome
Down's syndrome (Caused by trisomy 21)
Foreign body aspiration (FBA)

Goldenhar syndrome
Osteopetrosis
Pierre Robin syndrome
Respiratory failure
Snoring
Stridor
Treacher Collins syndrome
Wheezing

Epidemiology

Anatomic features of the immature airway, age-related developmental issues, and infectious disease susceptibilities lead to increased risk for severe respiratory compromise in pediatric patients.

The majority of cardiopulmonary arrests in the pediatric age group are precipitated by a primary respiratory cause.

- Primary cardiac arrest is rare in children. Hypoxemia and acidosis due to respiratory failure are the precursors of full arrest.

- The leading cause of preventable death in pediatric emergencies—both medical and trauma—is failure to adequately manage the airway.

- The airway is the key to success in pediatric resuscitation. Cardiovascular compromise can often be treated with oxygenation and ventilation alone.

Respiratory Failure

- Clinical state characterized by inadequate elimination of carbon dioxide (CO_2) and/or inadequate oxygenation of the blood.

- Seen as the end stage of respiratory distress of any cause or within adequate respiratory drive (ie, the patient with shallow respirations or apnea due to a head injury, seizure, or meningitis).

- Respiratory failure is often preceded by a "compensated" state characterized by respiratory distress: use of accessory muscles, retractions, tachypnea, and tachycardia.

- Clinical signs of respiratory failure reflect inadequate oxygen (O_2) delivery to the tissues and organs: decreased level of consciousness, tachycardia/bradycardia, weak proximal pulses, and poor skin perfusion.

Unique Features of the Pediatric Airway

- The tongue is relatively large in proportion to oral cavity, which is the most common cause of airway obstruction.

- Infants < 2 months of age are obligate nose breathers. Nasal obstruction, as with mucous or blood, may result in severe respiratory distress.

- The pediatric trachea is smaller and shorter than that of adults.
  - Smaller radius results in marked increase in resistance to air flow when edema or foreign is body present (Figure 11-1).

- The overall length of the trachea is much shorter. The trachea of a newborn is approximately 5 cm in length; and that of an 18-month old is approximately 7 cm. therefore; right mainstem intubation and accidental extubation are common.

- The larynx is relatively anterior and superior: C2 in the neonate, C3-4 in the child, C5-6 in the adult. Vocal cords may be difficult to visualize during laryngoscopy.

- The smallest diameter of the trachea is at the cricoid ring, below the cords, rather than at the vocal cords themselves.
  - Endotracheal (ET) tube size is dictated by the caliber of subglottic trachea.
  - Cuffed ET tubes are not used in children < 8years—the narrow subglottic region produces functional seal and prevents air leak.

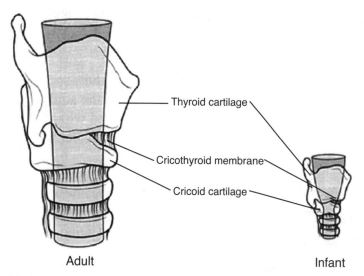

Adult   Infant

Figure 11-1 • Pediatric/adult airway comparison.
Reproduced with permission from Walls et al. *Manual of Emergency Airway Management.* 2nd ed. 2004. Lippincott Williams & Wilkins.

- Chest wall of infants relatively weak and unstable.
- Use of diaphragm leads to characteristic "see-saw" or abdominal breathing pattern.
- Intercostal, subcostal, and suprasternal retractions are prominent as work of breathing increases with airway obstruction or lung disease.
- Fatigue of respiratory muscles may lead to decreased respiratory effort as respiratory failure progresses.
- Immunologic immaturity leads to increased susceptibility to respiratory infections such as croup, epiglottitis, and bronchiolitis.
- Developmental immaturity leads to increased susceptibility to foreign body aspiration.

Auscultation of Lung Sounds

Abnormal lung sounds may be difficult to appreciate under noisy conditions in the field. If adequate auscultation is possible, the following sounds may help localize site of illness:

1. **Snoring**
   - Due to very proximal upper airway obstruction (tongue falling back against posterior pharynx).
2. **Stridor**
   - High-pitched noise heard on inspiration.
   - Due to upper airway obstruction (croup, epiglottitis, or foreign body).
3. **Wheezing**
   - Heard most commonly on expiration.
   - Indicates lower airway obstruction (asthma, bronchiolitis).
4. **Crackles**
   - Inspiratory noises; heard with parenchymal lung disease (pneumonia, bronchiolitis).

Common Pediatric Upper Airway Emergencies and Specific Management

The upper airway includes the oral and nasal cavities, pharynx, and trachea which runs all the way down to the level of the sternal notch.

Croup (Parainfluenza Virus)

1. Viral infection causing edema of vocal cords and adjacent trachea. Results in partial upper airway obstruction.
2. Accounts for approximately 90% of infectious upper airway problems in children.
3. Occurs more commonly in winter.
4. Children 6 months to 3 years are most commonly affected.
5. Clinical syndrome consists of cold symptoms and fever for several days, followed by respiratory distress, stridor, and barking cough.
6. Symptoms are often worse at night.
7. Course is subacute and respiratory failure is rare.

Croup Management

1. Cool, humidified air tends to alleviate obstruction associated with croup. Nebulized saline with no medication added can also be used to provide a cool watervapor to help reduce inflammation and swelling in croup.
2. Racemic epinephrine 2.25% solution for inhalation:
   - Dose: 0.5 cc in 4.5 cc NS nebulized.
   - Administration of racemic epinephrine in field commits the child to hospitalization due to rebound effect or a lengthy observation in the ED.
3. Cardiac monitoring required due to tachycardic effect and potential for arrhythmias.
4. In rare situations, the child with croup may present in respiratory failure unresponsive to BVM ventilation. Only in this case would endotracheal intubation be required. An ET tube one or two sizes smaller than normal should be used due to the swelling and inflammation of the trachea at the subglottic level.

Bacterial Upper Airway Infection and Epiglottitis Overview

- Life-threatening bacterial infection causing inflammation and edema of the epiglottis and/or adjacent structures above the larynx.

Swollen Epiglottis

- Epiglottitis is relatively rare due to widespread vaccination of infants against the bacteria *Haemophilus influenzae* type B but there are other causes of upper airway infection.

- Typically, more common in winter, but occurs year round.
- Children are usually older than 12 months.
- Onset is abrupt, with rapid progression to severe airway obstruction over hours.
- Fever, often up to 104°F, 40°C is generally the first sign and is present in almost every case.
- Sore throat or pain with swallowing usually present.
- As disease progresses, difficulty swallowing may lead to drooling and refusal to take fluids.
- Late in course, children may exhibit postural preference, which is assuming a seated position with jaw thrust forward—the "sniffing position"–to maximize air entry.
- Stridor may be present, but will not have the barking cough that is common with croup.
- Children tend to be very quiet and anxious.
- Complete obstruction and respiratory arrest will occur if definitive therapy not undertaken expeditiously. May be precipitated by agitation.

Bacterial Upper Airway Infection and Epiglottitis Management

- Minimize interventions if the child is conscious and maintaining their own airway.
- Instrumentation of oral cavity with an endotracheal blade or suction catheter may precipitate complete obstruction by laryngospasm.
- Administer 100% humidified O_2 via blow-by, as tolerated.
- Invasive procedures, such as IV placement, should not be performed unless lengthy transport is anticipated.
- If child loses consciousness, becomes apneic, or develops persistent central cyanosis despite administration of 100% O_2, positive pressure ventilation is required.
- Most children with epiglottitis can be ventilated with a bag-valve-mask.
- Excellent mask seal and high inspiratory pressures are required.
- Use a two-person BVM technique and override pop-off valve.
- If BVM ventilation is unsuccessful, attempt intubation using an ET one or two sizes smaller than anticipated for age.

- Chest compression by second rescuer may force a bubble of air through glottis and assist in identifying the cords.
- Aim the ET tube for the bubble of air.
- If patient cannot be intubated, needle cricothyroidotomy should be attempted. (See section later in chapter regarding cricothyroidotomy.)

What Went Wrong?

The occurrence of epiglottitis has decreased dramatically in the United States since the *Haemophilus influenzae* type B (*Hib*) vaccine became a routine childhood immunization in the 1980s.

Foreign Body Aspiration Overview (FBA)

- Common complication of childhood.
- Ages at highest risk: 6 months to 5 years > 90% of pediatric deaths due to foreign body aspiration occur in children < 5 years old; 65% in infants (see Figure 11-2).

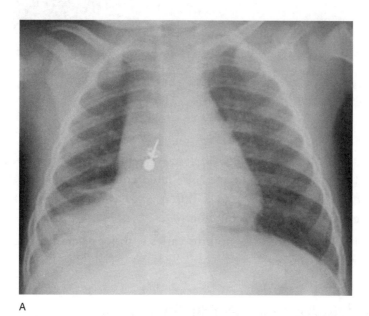

A

Figure 11-2 • A. Postero anterior and (B) lateral chest radiographs showing radiopaque bronchial foreign body. Reproduced with permission from Tintinalli JE, Stapczynski JS, Cline DM, Ma OJ, Cydulka RK, Meckler GD, eds. *Tintinalli's Emergency Medicine: A Comprehensive Study Guide.* 7th ed. 2011. New York: Copyright © McGraw-Hill Education. All rights reserved.

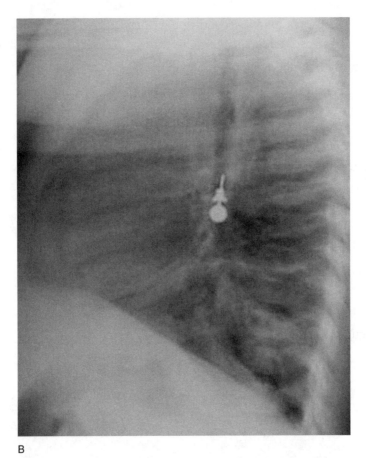

B

Figure 11-2 • *(Continued)*

- Diagnosis suspected in any previously well, afebrile child with sudden onset respiratory distress and associated coughing, choking, stridor, or wheezing. Less than 50% of children will have history of witnessed or suspected foreign body aspiration.
- Severity and nature of symptoms varies with location of foreign body in respiratory tract.

Foreign Body Aspiration Management

- Minimize field interventions if the child is conscious and maintaining their own airway.
- Administer 100% O_2 as tolerated.

- Mouth sweeps should not be attempted unless foreign body is visible and child's cooperation can be assured. Blind sweeps may lead to impaction of foreign body in glottis and complete obstruction.

- If wheezing is present and foreign body is in a small airway then attempts to dislodge should not be undertaken in field.

- Tracheal foreign body causing complete obstruction, loss of consciousness, central cyanosis unresponsive to 100% O_2, or gasping respirations; perform chest compressions.

What Went Wrong?

According to the 2010 AHA Guidelines in an unresponsive choking pediatric patient, begin cardiopulmonary resuscitation (CPR) (start with chest compressions first) with one added step. Each time you open the airway to perform ventilations, you should look for the obstruction in the back of the throat. If the object is seen and can easily be removed, remove it.

- If the foreign body is not expelled by the maneuver described above, perform direct laryngoscopy and remove visible foreign body with pediatric Magill forceps.

- If foreign body is not visualized, attempt to intubate and push foreign body into lower airway.

- If child cannot be intubated, needle cricothyroidotomy should be attempted.

Common Lower Airway/Pulmonary Emergencies

Asthma Overview

Asthma is a disease characterized by hyper-reactive small airways and reversible obstruction of those airways. There are three components of obstruction:

1. Bronchoconstriction
2. Mucosal edema
3. Increased secretions

Asthma is the most common pediatric chronic disease. Attacks are precipitated by variety of causes—infections, allergies, cold, exercise, and stress.

- Characterized by wheezing, cough, and increased work of breathing.

- Children in severe distress may assume "tripod" position, leaning forward on hands to facilitate use of accessory muscles of respiration.

- With severe obstruction air entry may be so compromised that wheezing disappears, this is called a "quiet chest" signaling impending respiratory failure.
- Severity of symptoms varies widely from mild distress to respiratory arrest.

Bronchiolitis Overview

Bronchiolitis is a viral infection causing obstruction of lower airways and symptom complex similar to asthma.

- Most common in children < 2 years.
- Epidemics occur in winter months.
- The respiratory syncytial virus (RSV) is responsible for over 50% of the cases.

Clinical Fact

RSV is a very common pediatric illness. It's seen more often than the seasonal flu. According to the CDC, the RSV season in the United States begins in the fall, peaks in the winter, and ends late winter or early spring. The exact timing varies year to year and geographic area.

- Characterized by diffuse crackles, wheezing, and increased work of breathing, with tachypnea, nasal flaring, and retractions.
- Apnea is a complication seen primarily in young infants.
- Infants with pre-existing cardiopulmonary disease have an increased incidence of death related to RSV infection.
- Unlike asthma, obstruction is poorly responsive to bronchodilator medications.

Asthma/Bronchiolitis Management

- Administer supplemental O_2.
- A severe asthma attack can be treated with bronchodilator drugs.

Nebulized Therapy

- May be better tolerated than IM epinephrine, especially by older children.
- May be administered by blow-by to infants too young to accept mouthpiece.
- Sympathetic side effects (tachycardia, tremor, nausea) less pronounced than seen with epinephrine.

- Albuterol (Proventil), 0.5% or 5 mg/mL solution for inhalation can be given as follows:

  - < 15 kg: 2.5 or 5.0 mg (0.5-1.0 mL) diluted in 3 mL of normal saline, nebulized. May repeat every 20 to 30 minutes × 2 or use continuously in critical patients.

  - > 15 kg: 5 to 10 mg (1-2 mL) diluted in 3 mL of normal saline, nebulized. May repeat every 20 to 30 minutes × 2 or use continuously in critical patients.

Albuterol Metered-Dose Inhaler (MDI)

Four to eight puffs every 20 minutes, administer with mask or spacer device.

- Bronchodilator drugs may cause tachycardia and arrhythmias.
- Perform continuous cardiac monitoring
- If a wheezing child cannot tolerate nebulized or inhaled drug therapy or is not moving enough air to inhale the drug properly, give IM epinephrine. Epinephrine: 0.01 cc/kg 1:1,000 solution IM in the deltoid muscle or anterior thigh of infants; maximum dose = 0.3 cc; may repeat 20 to 30 minutes × 2.

What Went Wrong?

Status Asthmaticus

This is an acute exacerbation of asthma that remains unresponsive to initial treatment with bronchodilators. It ranges from mild to severe and presents with bronchospasm, airway inflammation, mucous plugging, difficulty breathing, CO_2 retention, hypoxemia, and respiratory failure.

- Consider positive pressure ventilation with a BVM and ET intubation only if the child is in respiratory failure and has failed to respond to high-flow O_2 and maximal bronchodilator therapy.

Bronchopulmonary Dysplasia (BPD)

- It is seen in infants who are born prematurely. It is an example of a chronic disorder that develops in premature infants as a result of the therapies used to treat their immature lungs. Typically seen in premature babies born more than 10 weeks before their due date and whose weight is less than 2 pounds (1,000 g) at birth.
- Prolonged exposure to high O_2 concentrations, endotracheal intubation, ventilator pressures, and fluid overload damage the pulmonary tree. These infants are medically fragile and susceptible to respiratory infections.

- These infants normally expend considerable energy to breathe and are frequently on home O_2 and multiple medications. In addition, they may have delay in normal growth and development due to their prematurity or have significant disabilities such as cerebral palsy, mental retardation, deafness, and blindness.
- This is characterized by chronic respiratory distress. Signs include retractions, crackles, and wheezing.
- There is a high mortality rate in the first year of life and parents are often extremely anxious.
- These are medically fragile children who have minimum respiratory reserve and can be at risk from even a minor infection. They may decompensate quickly and may require increased O_2, airway ventilation interventions, and bronchodilator medications.

Prediction of Difficult Airways in Children

As in adults, difficult airways in children may or may not be anticipated. Some forms of difficult airway, either difficult bag-mask ventilation or difficult intubation, may be anticipated in the following congenital or acquired disorders.

Congenital Disorders Associated with Difficult Airways in Children

Congenital disorders are rare and include genetic and chromosomal disorders. Conditions typically associated with difficult airways can be divided into those conditions associated with hypoplasia of the mandible, hypoplasia of the midface, or associated with a large tongue (macroglossia).

Syndromes Associated with Mandibular Hypoplasia

Pierre Robin Syndrome
Features (see Figure 11-3a):

- Micrognathia (undersized jaw)
- Glossoptosis (backward displacement of the tongue)
- U-shaped cleft palate
- Associated cardiac abnormalities—pulmonary stenosis, patent ductus arteriosus, patent foramen ovale

These patients may require a tracheostomy early in infancy if the glossoptosis or micrognathia causes airway obstruction with apnea. Cleft palate repair is usually performed at around 9 months of age.

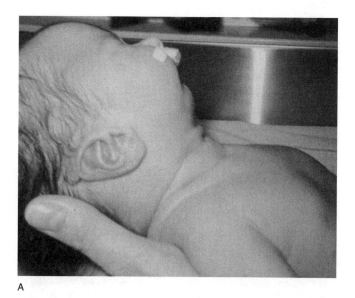

A

Figure 11-3a • Pierre Robin syndrome.
Reproduced with permission from Fuster V, Walsh RA, Harrington RA, eds. *Hurst's The Heart.*
13th ed. 2011. New York: Copyright © McGraw-Hill Education. All rights reserved.

Airway problem:

- Difficult bag-valve mask ventilation (poor mask fitting) and intubation.

Treacher Collins Syndrome

Features (see Figure 11-3b):

- Bilateral malar and mandibular hypoplasia associated with obstructive sleep apnea (OSA) or airway obstruction while awake.
- Malformation of external pinna and ear canal.

Airway problem:

- Difficult intubation, which may be worsened by corrective surgery

Goldenhar Syndrome

Features:

- Asymmetrical malar, maxillary, and mandibular hypoplasia
- Auricular and ocular defects
- Cardiac defects—ventricular septal defect or tetralogy of Fallot

Airway problems:

- Maintaining an airway, laryngoscopy, and intubation
- Mouth opening has cleft-like extension on the affected side—mask fit may be a problem.

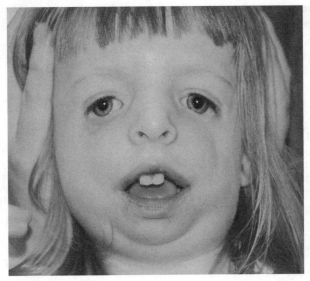

B

Figure 11-3b • Treacher Collins syndrome.
Reproduced with permission from Brunicardi FC, Andersen DK, Billiar TR, Dunn DL, Hunter JG, Matthews JB, Pollock RE, eds. *Schwartz's Principles of Surgery*. 9th ed. 2010. New York: Copyright © McGraw-Hill Education. All rights reserved.

Syndromes Associated with Mid-Face Hypoplasia

Crouzon Syndrome

Features:

- Premature fusion of multiple cranial sutures
- Maxillary hypoplasia
- Orbital proptosis
- Hypertelorism (widely spaced eyes)

Airway problem:

- Difficult facemask ventilation, intubation usually not difficult

Apert Syndrome

Features (see Figure 11-3c):

- Irregular premature fusion of multiple cranial sutures
- Midface hypoplasia/hypertelorism
- Syndactyly (two or more digits are fused together)
- Possible choanal stenosis

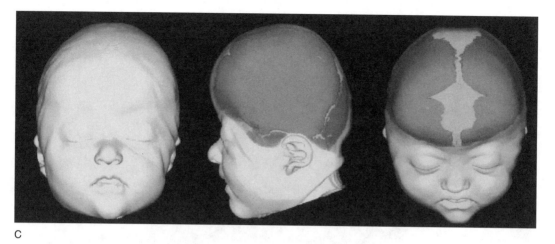

c

Figure 11-3c • Apert syndrome.
Reproduced with permission from Rudolph CD, Rudolph A, Lister GE, First L, Gershon A, eds. *Rudolph's Pediatrics*. 22nd ed. 2011. New York: Copyright © McGraw-Hill Education. All rights reserved.

- Progressive calcification of hands, feet, and cervical spine
- 10% incidence of cardiac defects/genitourinary anomalies

Airway problem:

- Bag mask ventilation may be difficult but intubation is usually straightforward. A smaller size ET may be required.

Conditions Associated with Limited Neck Movement

Down's Syndrome (Caused by Trisomy 21)

Features (see Figure 11-4):

- Macroglossia
- Atlanto-axial subluxation
- Cardiac anomalies, particularly atrioventricular septal defect
- May be difficult to perform positive pressure ventilation via bag-valve-mask ventilation due to macroglossia. In children with atlanto-axial instability, the EMS providers will need to maintain in-line neck stabilization.

Osteopetrosis

Features:

- Bones become increasingly dense
- Limited mouth opening
- Limited neck movement

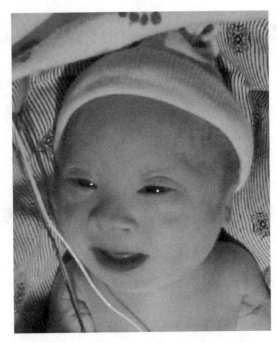

Figure 11-4 • Down's syndrome.
Reproduced with permission from Cunningham FG, Leveno KJ, Bloom SL, Hauth JC, Rouse DJ, Spong CY, eds. *Williams Obstetrics*. 23rd ed. New York: McGraw-Hill; 2010. (Photograph courtesy of Dr. Charles P. Read and Dr. Lewis Weber.)

Airway problem:

- Difficult bag-valve-mask ventilation and intubation.

Tracheal Abnormalities

Children with laryngeal or tracheal abnormalities present difficulties with passage of a tracheal tube through the larynx, although visualization of the larynx may not be difficult.

Congenital Subglottic Stenosis

Features:

- Incomplete recanalization of the laryngotracheal airway during the third month of gestation.

Clinical presentation: These children present with recurrent stridor that becomes worse with upper respiratory infection or as the child grows. Differential diagnosis is recurrent croup.

Airway problem:

- Difficult intubation (laryngoscopy usually normal) requiring smaller size endotracheal tube.

Acquired Subglottic Stenosis

Caused by trauma to the subglottic structure secondary to endotracheal intubation, but may also be due to a foreign body, infection, or chemical irritation. Scar tissue is formed when healing takes place that may contract circumferentially to produce narrowing or severe stenosis. As for children with congenital subglottic stenosis, these children present with stridor that may become worse with upper respiratory infection.

Direct Laryngoscopy

The first attempt at laryngoscopy should be performed under optimal conditions, with the head and neck placed in the optimal position (neck flexed, head extended). Neonates have a large occiput and may benefit from a shoulder roll (Figure 11-5a, b, c); a pillow should not be used for infants and small children, as this tends to flex the neck too much. The patient should be well oxygenated.

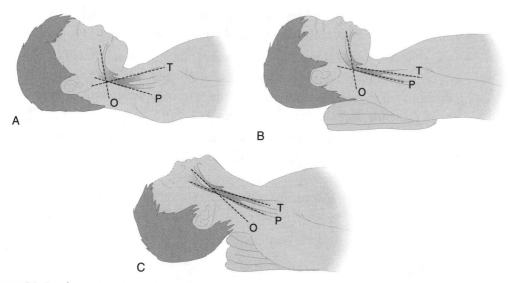

Figure 11-5a, b, c • Head positions during intubation.
Reproduced with permission from Tintinalli JE, Stapczynski JS, Cline DM, Ma OJ, Cydulka RK, Meckler GD, eds. *Tintinalli's Emergency Medicine: A Comprehensive Study Guide.* 7th ed. 2011. New York: Copyright © McGraw-Hill Education. All rights reserved.

The pediatric larynx is more anterior and cephalic than an adult, and external laryngeal manipulation may be useful to obtain a good view at laryngoscopy.

A Miller blade laryngoscope is recommended in neonates due to their large U-shaped floppy epiglottis, using the blade to pick up the epiglottis. If muscle relaxants are not used, take care that you do not provoke laryngospasm during manipulation of the airway; if muscle relaxants are used, an adequate depth of paralysis must be maintained at all times, and the relative merits of a short-acting nondepolarizing muscle relaxant should be considered. There are currently no published algorithms for managing difficult intubation in the pediatric population. In line with adult patients, it is suggested that total intubation attempts should be limited to three as the pediatric airway is very susceptible to trauma, and a *can't intubate* situation may develop quickly into *can't intubate* and *can't ventilate* if the airway becomes edematous. Children and infants will desaturate more quickly than adults, and the child must be ventilated between each intubation attempt to maintain oxygenation as well as an adequate level of sedation. Endotracheal intubation should be attempted only by highly-trained medical providers who maintain their skill levels through experience or frequent retraining. Demonstration of skill on infant and pediatric manikins should be an integral part of classroom training.

What Went Wrong?

"Can't intubate, can't ventilate" requires emergency techniques which include either needle cricothyroidotomy or a surgical cricothyroidotomy.

- Indications for field intubation of the pediatric patient include: inability to oxygenate/ventilate via bag-valve-mask; prolonged transport time and ongoing need for assisted ventilation; need for tracheal suctioning; need for access route for resuscitation medications.

- Risks of intubation are similar in pediatric and adult patients. Infants become hypoxemic more quickly than adults when deprived of O_2. EMS personnel must be especially conscious of duration of intubation attempts in pediatric patients and ensure adequate preoxygenation via BVM prior to each attempt.

Equipment

Safe and successful intubation requires age-appropriate equipment.

- It is easier to intubate an infant using a Miller laryngoscope blade. A Miller or Macintosh blade may be used in children, according to paramedic's experience and degree of comfort with the equipment. Blade size is chosen according to age.

- Endotracheal tubes:
  - Tube size is dictated by age. Size can be approximated by choosing tube equal to diameter of child's little finger or nostril. Tube of one size bigger and one size smaller should be at hand.
  - Cuffed tubes are not used in children under 8 years of age, due to differences in airway anatomy. In these children, the cricoid ring is the narrowest portion of the airway and acts as a natural cuff.
- Intubation of infants, using small floppy tubes, may be facilitated by use of a stylet to guide the tube through the cords. Care should be taken that tip of stylet is at least a centimeter proximal to the tip of the tube (to avoid tracheal damage).
- Use of a Broselow™ Pediatric Emergency tape has proven to be very accurate in determining patient weight, which will help reduce drug dosage errors.

Intubation Drugs

The use of neuromuscular blockade drugs will be dictated by local protocol for pediatric patients.

Commonly used agents include succinylcholine and pancuronium. The use of succinylcholine in young children, especially with repeat doses, may be associated with profound bradycardia. For that reason, pretreatment with atropine is recommended when succinylcholine is to be used.

Doses:

1. Atropine: 0.02 mg/kg IV or ET with a minimum dose of 0.1 mg
2. Succinylcholine: 1 mg/kg IV or 4 mg/kg IM
3. Pancuronium: 0.1 mg/kg IV

Intubation Technique

Cricoid pressure (Sellick maneuver) is sometimes used to enhance visualization of cords, which may be difficult due to their anterior placement in young children.

1. Cricoid pressure should be used with caution in young infants where it may cause tracheal compression/obstruction due to incomplete formation of cartilaginous tracheal rings.

2. Young children become hypoxic rapidly. Limit each intubation attempt to 20 seconds, and preoxygenate with 100% O_2. Heart rate must be monitored during intubation attempts, as hypoxia rapidly leads to bradycardia in children.

3. Do not force a tight tube. The narrowest part of the child's airway is below the cords.

4. Watch as tube is advanced, as the airway is short and mainstem bronchus intubation is a common complication. The tip of an uncuffed tube should be 2 or 3 cm below cords. Pediatric tubes have three sets of rings marking their distal end or a dark tip (Figure 11-6). If the second ring is at the level of the cords, the tube is in mid-tracheal position. Tube position can also be assessed by centimeter marking at the lips.

Confirming Endotracheal Tube Placement

Once you have the child intubated, hold the tube firmly at the level of the lip and evaluate placement:

Primary Tube Confirmation:

- Provide positive-pressure ventilation and observe for bilateral, symmetrical chest rise. Remove the tube if there is no chest rise with ventilation.

- Listen for gurgling over the epigastrium which indicates esophageal intubation. Breath sounds should be absent over the upper abdomen but in a small child it may be transmitted sounds from the lungs. Remove the tube if you also see noticeable gastric distention with ventilation.

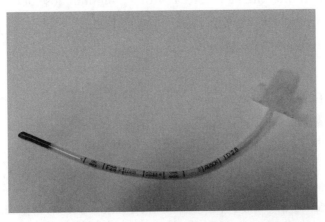

Figure 11-6 • Photo of the distal end of a 2.0 tube. Photo by: Peter A. DiPrima Jr.

- Listen for equal breath sounds bilaterally over the peripheral lung fields and in the axillary areas indicating proper tube placement in the trachea. If breath sounds are equal, secure the tube. If sounds are louder on the right side, then slowly pull back the ET tube until breath sounds are equal as it may be in the right main\stem bronchus.

- Observe the child for signs of clinical improvement such as improved color, perfusion, and O_2 saturation.

Secondary Tube Confirmation

Secondary tube placement confirmation should be done with an end-tidal CO_2 detector or capnography.

Securing the Endotracheal Tube

- Secure tube carefully. The infant or young child's airway is short and a small amount of displacement can lead to mainstem bronchus intubation or accidental extubation, even if the tube was initially placed correctly. Accidental extubation most commonly occurs during loading or unloading patients from ambulances or other transport vehicles or isolettes.

- In older children, it is preferred to secure the tube with a commercially made ET tube holder device of an appropriate size rather than tape.

- In younger children and infants with small tubes, taping to secure the tube is necessary:

  - Insert a correct-sized oral airway as a bite block, making sure not to compress the tube.

  - Cut two pieces of 1-inch wide tape approximately 6 inches in length. Cut or tear the pieces in half lengthwise for approximately 4 inches (leave a 2-inch length of tape that remains the full width) (see Figure 11-7a).

  - Apply the intact piece of adhesive tape to the cheek and adhere to one length of the torn portion across the upper lip. (see Figure 11-7b)

  - Wrap the second length of the torn portion around the tube at least two to three times (see Figure 11-7c).

  - Apply the second strip in a similar fashion from the opposite direction (see Figure 11-7d).

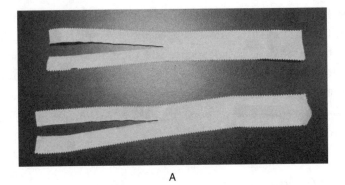

A

Figure 11-7a • Photo by: Peter A. DiPrima Jr.

- Intubated patients should have a C collar on to protect the ET tube placement during transport. (If a cervical doesn't fit the patient towel rolls can be used.)
- Document the location of the ET tube at the lip or gum line. Reassess tube position continuously.

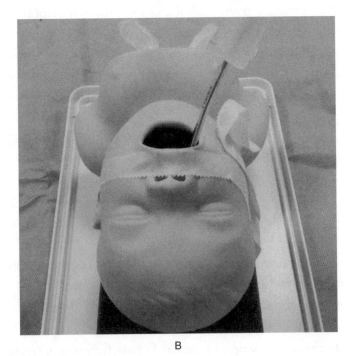

B

Figure 11-7b • Photo by: Peter A. DiPrima Jr.

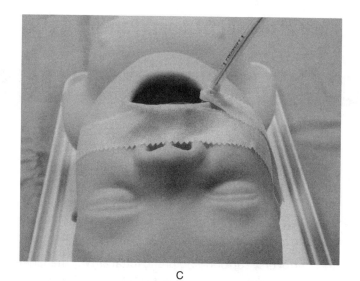

C

Figure 11-7c • Photo by: Peter A. DiPrima Jr.

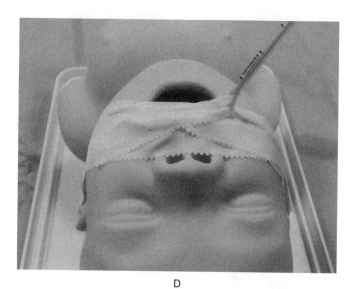

D

Figure 11-7d • Photo by: Peter A. DiPrima Jr.

Airway Management of the Adult Trauma Patient

LEARNING OBJECTIVES

At the end of this chapter, you will be able to:

● Understand the priorities of trauma management.

● Be able to rapidly and accurately assess a trauma patients airway.

● Be able to resuscitate and stabilize trauma patients.

● Discuss the key elements of the neurological examination in patients with severe traumatic brain injury.

● Present the controversy surrounding prehospital airway management of patients with severe traumatic brain injury (TBI).

● Discuss indications for ICP monitoring.

● Discuss strategies in managing increased ICP.

The absolute priority in the initial resuscitation of any trauma is to secure a patent airway and provide adequate ventilation. Even under the best of conditions, securing a patent airway may be challenging in a trauma patient, but it is particularly difficult in patients with traumatic injuries to the airway, in whom complex airway management techniques maybe required.

Indication for RSI of the Acute Trauma Patient

- Trauma patients with GCS < 8
- Significant facial trauma with poor airway control
- Airway obstruction
- Closed head injury or hemorrhagic CVA
- Burn patients with airway involvement and inevitable airway loss
- Class 3-4 hemorrhagic shock
- Failure to maintain adequate oxygenation ($PaO_2 < 60$ despite 100% FiO_2)
- Paralysis due to high spinal cord injury
- Need for positive pressure ventilation
- Blunt chest trauma with compromised ventilatory effort
- Mandibular fractures with loss of airway muscular support

Drugs Used in Managing the Airway of the Trauma Patient

Sedatives

Midazolam (Versed): Dose: 0.1 mg/kg

- Strong benzodiazepine
- Rapid onset (1 or 2 minutes) and short duration (20 minutes)
- Has an amnesic affect, is used as an anticonvulsant and muscle relaxant
- Slight decrease in blood pressure and increase in pulse rate.
- No increase in ICP.

Etomidate: Dose: 0.3 mg/kg

- Nonbarbiturate, nonnarcotic sedative-hypnotic induction agent.
- Good agent in multisystem trauma patient because it evokes minimal change in HR and CO compared to other sedatives. (Ideal agent in any patient in shock including cardiogenic and septic shock.)
- Decreases ICP and IOP during intubation.
- Rapid onset (< 1 minute) and short acting (5 minutes).
- Vomiting, especially when combined with a narcotic.

Thiopental: Dose: 3 to 5 mg/kg

- Ultra-short acting barbiturate sedative.
- Onset 30 to 40 seconds and last 10 minutes.
- Does not cause increase in ICP but can cause severe hypotension, therefore avoid in multitrauma patients.
- Can also induce bronchospasm.

Fentanyl: Dose: 3 to 5 µg/kg

- Narcotic.
- Little or no histamine release.
- Rarely causes hypotension.
- Consider in head-injured patients as a premedication to prevent increase in ICP (blunts pressor response).
- Rapid injection may cause chest wall rigidity.
- Onset in 2 minutes with 30 to 40 minute duration.

Paralytic Agents

Vecuronium: nondepolarizing agent. 1/3 more potent and pancuronium and duration of action is 1/3 to ½ as long (25-40 minutes versus pancuronium which last 2-3 hours)

- Onset 2 to 3 minutes.
- Dose does not cause the degree of tachycardia seen with pancuronium.
- No histamine release.
- Defasciculating dose: 0.01 mg/kg.
- Paralytic dose: 0.1 mg/kg.

Succinylcholine: depolarizing agent, which causes muscle fasciculations which can be prevented by pretreatment with a nondepolarizing neuromuscular agent.

- Rapid onset (30-60 seconds) with short duration of action (5-7 minutes).

Dose:

- Adult: 1.5 mg/kg
- Pediatric (<10 y/o): 2.0 mg/kg

Contraindications:

- Burns > 7 days old
- Extensive crush injuries > 7 days old
- Paraplegia > 7 days old
- Narrow-angle glaucoma
- Neuromuscular diseases, such as:
  - Guillain-Barre, Myasthenia Gravis, multiple sclerosis, muscular dystrophy, Parkinson's disease
- Others susceptible to increased potassium: renal failure (no real evidence that RSI increases K^+)
- Rhabdomyolysis

Rocuronium: nondepolarizing agent

- Onset < 1 minute
- Duration 20 to 30 minutes

Dose: 0.9 to 1.2 mg/kg

Adjunctive Drug Therapy

Atropine: succinylcholine will cause bradycardia in infants and children. Therefore, they should be premedicated with atropine. Also pretreat any adult who is already bradycardic. Children < 8 years. Dose: 0.01 mg/kg up to 0.5 mg (minimum dose of 0.1 mg).

Lidocaine: Dose: 1.5 mg/kg

Some studies recommend intravenous lidocaine to blunt the pressor response of increased pulse, increased blood pressure, increased intracranial pressure, and increased intraocular pressure associated with intubation, its usefulness is controversial. However, because a single dose of lidocaine is unlikely to cause harm, it seems reasonable to use in the patient who has a known or suspected head injury.

1. Should be administered 2 to 3 minutes prior to intubation.

Procedure

1. Preoxygenation with 100% O_2 for 3 to 5 minutes via NRB mask (or 3 vital capacity breaths, avoid BVM if possible).
2. Secure IVs, ECG, pulse oximeter.
3. Prepare intubation equipment: ETT with stylet, suction, BVM, laryngoscope.
4. Premedication:
   - Lidocaine (head injury) 1.5 mg/kg
   - Vecuronium (defasciculating dose) 0.01 mg/kg
   - Versed 0.1 mg/kg
   - Atropine (pediatrics) 0.01 mg/kg
   - Etomidate 0.3 mg/kg
5. Administer succinylcholine 1.5 mg/kg (pediatrics: 2.0 mg/kg)
6. Wait 30 to 60 seconds, place ETT.
7. Confirm ETT placement by: listening for bilateral breath sounds, chest rise and fall, tube fogging, and positive $EtCO_2$. Final confirmation should be by CXR (in hospital).
8. Secure ETT.

Initial Management of Head Injuries

Brain injury is the most common cause of death in trauma. Brain injury is divided into primary and secondary forms. Primary brain injury, which occurs immediately upon impact, can be reduced only through prevention initiatives. Secondary brain injury, which ensues within hours to days later, results from a cascade of cellular events (intracellular calcium, cell membrane permeability changes, depletion of cellular energy, free radical generation, cell signaling molecules) that harms or even destroys neuronal tissue in and around the site of the primary injury.

Secondary injury is exacerbated by four major factors:

1. Hypoxia

2. Hypotension

3. Hypercarbia

4. Intracranial hypertension

Additional factors which also affect secondary brain injury include hypocapnea, hyperthermia, glucose imbalance, acute hypo-osmolarity, electrolyte imbalance, anemia, acid–base disorders, and coagulopathy. Since secondary brain injury is a major contributor to brain injury mortality and has a negative effect on neurologic outcome, paramedics must work diligently to identify and treat causative factors. Airway maintenance, ventilation, CO_2 control, and restoration of circulating volume using isotonic fluid are essential initial treatments. SBP < 90 and SaO_2< 90% must be strictly avoided in head-injured patients.

Critical Care Paramedicine

During interfacility transports, ICP monitoring is indicated in salvageable patients with GCS ≤ 8 and an abnormal CT scan. Some evidence also suggests ICP monitoring is indicated in patients with a normal CT if GCS ≤ 8 and age > 40, SBP< 90 or bi- or unilateral posturing. Though older devices were subarachnoid, subdural, or epidural, modern ICP monitors are intraparenchymal or intraventricular. ICP monitoring guides therapy, and if an intraventricular catheter is in place, permits drainage. ICP monitoring also predicts outcome, as patients who respond the therapy for intracranial hypertension have a more favorable outcome. Normal ICP is 0 to 15 mm Hg. Therapy should be initiated to lower ICP when it reaches 20 mm Hg. More important than ICP is cerebral perfusion pressure (CPP), the difference between MAP and ICP (CPP = MAP-ICP). CPP < 50 mm Hg must be strictly avoided and recommended CPP is 50 to 70 mm Hg, though optimal CPP is unproven. CPP may be increased by lowering ICP or by raising MAP. ICP may be lowered by removal of noxious stimuli and adequate sedation. Morphine is sedative and analgesic without increasing ICP. Midazolam may reduce MAP and raise ICP. Propofol is the recommended sedative agent in brain injured patients because it lowers ICP. MAP can be increased by use of alpha-adrenergic agents.

Alternative measures for brain oxygenation include jugular venous oxygen saturation (SjO_2) and brain tissue partial pressure of oxygen ($PbrO_2$). If measured, interventions to increase cerebral oxygenation when SjO_2 drops below 50% and/or $PbrO_2$ drops below 15 mm Hg. Mannitol is a hyperosmolar plasma expander that also functions as an osmotic diuretic. Mannitol expands plasma volume, reduces blood viscosity, increases cerebral blood flow, and O_2 delivery and because of its osmotic effects may reduce brain water and secondary brain injury. Mannitol (0.25 g-1 g/kg) can be used to lower ICP based upon clinical signs alone (herniation or progressive neurologic decline) or ICP monitoring. Paramedics must maintain adequate intravascular volume in the face of mannitol therapy, and should follow doctor orders written prior to or during transport.

Hyperventilation has theoretical benefits in lowering PCO_2 and thus cerebral blood volume which lowers ICP. Hypocapnea can, however, produce cerebral ischemia and recent data indicate that hypocapnea may be more harmful than hypercapnea. Moreover, prolonged hyperventilation is probably ineffective because adaptation occurs and cerebral blood flow returns to baseline. Current guidelines for CO_2 control are to achieve a $PCO_2 = 35$ and avoid hyperventilation to $PCO_2 < 35$ mm Hg for the first 24 hours postinjury. Hyperventilation may be used as a temporizing measure only in cases of refractory intracranial hypertension.

Additional treatments for severe traumatic brain injury include barbiturates which are recommended for refractory intracranial hypertension in hemodynamically stable patients. Hemodynamic instability is side effect of this therapy. Steroids are contraindicated for the treatment of traumatic brain injury. Anticonvulsants (phenytoin) may be used to prevent early post-traumatic seizures and therapy duration is ≈ 7 days. Prophylactic antibiotics are not recommended for indwelling ICP monitors. DVT prophylaxis is recommended in patients with TBI, with compression devices initially and progressing to anticoagulants.

Prehospital Treatment

Ensure patent airway while maintaining cervical spine precautions (endotracheal intubation using RSI protocol) if necessary.

- Ventilate patient with 100% O_2. Keep $PaO_2 > 60$ mm Hg (Sat > 90%).
- Keep $EtCO_2$ 30-35 mm Hg during transport.
- Establish adequate IV access.
- Maintain mean arterial pressure (MAP) > 90.

- Mannitol may be given with ingoing signs if neurologic deterioration:
  - motor score< 3
  - decreasing motor score
  - lateralizing motor findings
  - pupillary changes (dilation or sluggish reactivity)
- Sedation/neuromuscular blockade can be useful in optimizing transport of head injured patient. Both treatments interfere with neurologic examination and should be avoided if possible.
  - reassess neurologic status frequently.
  - transfer should not be delayed for diagnostic testing.
  - steroids have not been found to be of benefit to the head-injured patient and are not recommended as therapy for severe head injury.

Initial Resuscitation of the Head-Injured Patient

- Insure patent airway (endotracheal intubation is indicated in patients with GCS < 8).
- Maintain cervical spine immobilization.
- Maintain MAP > 90 throughout patient course in attempt to maintain cerebral perfusion pressure (CPP) 50 to 70 mm Hg. Insure adequate volume repletion before adding vasopressors (CVP > 12).
- Maintain adequate circulating volume:
  - Normal saline (NS) is the recommended solution for the TBI patient.
  - monitor for signs of diabetes insipidus.
  - place Foley catheter, as dictated by local protocol.
  - prophylactic anti-convulsants may be indicated.

Emergency Airway Evaluation of the Burn Patient

LEARNING OBJECTIVES

At the end of this chapter, you will be able to:

- Describe the initial evaluation and assessment of the burned patient.
- List the different types of burns and their distinguishing characteristics.
- Name the potential for comorbid injuries in inhalational injury.
- List the basic principles of burn management.

Stabilization

Maintain airway—the supraglottic airway is extremely susceptible to obstruction from edema as a result of exposure to superheated air. Assess for clinical signs of inhalation injury:

- Facial burns/singeing of the eyebrows and nasal hairs (see Figure 11-8).
- Carbonaceous sputum and acute inflammatory changes in the oropharynx, raspy voice.
- History of impaired mentation and/or confinement in a burning environment.
- Assess for toxic inhalation, or carbon monoxide poisoning.

Respiratory complications caused by smoke inhalation, burns, and their treatment epitomize the challenges which confront EMT and paramedics caring for burn patients. Smoke inhalation injury and its sequelae impose demands upon the paramedics who play a central role in its clinical prehospital management.

What Went Wrong?

Transport medicine: upper airway injury that results in obstruction during the first12 hours after insult is caused by direct thermal injury as well as chemical irritation.

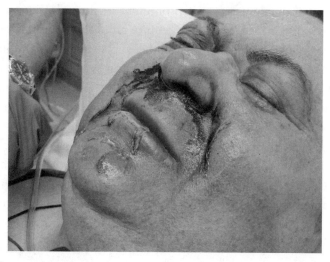

Figure 11-8 • Facial burns.
Reproduced with permission from Knoop KJ, Stack LB, Storrow AB, Thurman RJ, eds. *The Atlas of Emergency Medicine*. 3rd ed. 2010. New York: Copyright © McGraw-Hill Education. All rights reserved. (Photo contributor: Chan W. Park, MD.)

The pathophysiologic changes in the parenchyma of the lungs that are associated with inhalation injury are not the result of direct thermal injury. Only steam, with a heat-carrying capacity many times that of dry air, is capable of overwhelming the extremely efficient heat-dissipatory capabilities of the upper airways. Nor is the carbonaceous material present in smoke directly responsible for damage, although it can serve as a carrier for other agents. Damage to the lung parenchyma is caused by the incomplete products of combustion. Many substances present in burning cotton are injurious, but the most important products are the aldehydes and oxides of sulphur and nitrogen. Burning polyvinylchloride (PVC) yields at least 75 potentially toxic compounds, including hydrochloric acid and carbon monoxide.

Carbon Monoxide

An invisible, odorless gas, carbon monoxide has a much stronger affinity for hemoglobin than does O_2, leading to a tremendous reduction in the oxygen-carrying capacity. The shortage of O_2 at the tissue level is made worse by a concomitant leftward shift of the oxyhemoglobin dissociation curve. The pathology of the upper and lower respiratory tract lesions is due to the formation of edema. Acute upper airway obstruction (UAO) occurs in approximately one-fifth to one-third of hospitalized burn victims with inhalation injury. A major hazard because of the possibility of rapid progression from mild pharyngeal edema to complete upper airway obstruction with asphyxia. The worsening of upper airway edema is most prominent in supraglottic structures. For patients with large surface burns that require rapid fluid administration, these changes may be accentuated. Burns of the neck, especially in children, can cause unyielding eschars that externally compress and obstruct the airway. Whenever UAO is suspected the most experienced paramedic in airway management should perform endotracheal intubation. Securing the endotracheal tube can be difficult due to the burn wound and the rapid swelling that occurs. Inhalation injury and associated major burns provide a challenge for health care workers who provide direct hands-on care. The technical and physiological problems, which complicate the respiratory management of these patients, require an orderly, systematic approach. Successful outcomes require careful attention to treatment priorities, protocols and meticulous attention to details.

Management

Airway: ensure patency and stability. Check for exposure to heat and thermal injury to the nose, mouth, face, and look for singed hair. Consider smoke involvement if soot is on the face and in the sputum, although smoke inhalation is possible without evidence of soot. When upper airway injury is suspected, elective intubation should be considered because progression of edema over the next 24 to 48 hours may make intubation difficult if not impossible.

Breathing: check for upper airway compromise, difficulty breathing, stridor, cough, retractions, and bilateral breath sounds. Administer 100% O_2 because of the likelihood of CO inhalation in fires.

The direct effects of inhalation injury are usually evident within the first 24 hours, although pulmonary dysfunction may result from complex hemodynamic and infectious complications associated with surface burns.

Circulation: patients whose injury involves cutaneous burns have ongoing circulatory derangements. Fluid loss through burned areas from intense inflammation with vasodilation and capillary leak or from the subsequent infectious complications necessitates large fluid volume resuscitation. Even minor errors in estimation of body surface area, burned surface area, fluid electrolyte, and protein requirements can produce profound hemodynamic and respiratory embarrassment.

Disability: patient responsiveness helps determine the ability to protect the airway and is also an excellent indicator of adequacy of resuscitation.

Expose: check all body areas for additional burns and injuries.

Airway Management in Pregnancy

LEARNING OBJECTIVES

At the end of this chapter, you will be able to:

- Recognize and evaluate the differences in the obstetrical patient.
- Review the anatomical and physiological changes that occur during pregnancy that cause difficult airway management.
- Management of the pregnant patient.

Introduction

Several factors tend to evoke apprehension in even the most competent paramedic when dealing with the airway in a pregnant woman. The most important reasons being pregnancy-related altered anatomy and physiology impacting airway management and the urgent nature of obstetric patients lead to limited time for adequate preparation, and the potential risk of impacting both mother and fetus. Failed tracheal intubation is well documented in the obstetric population, with an incidence eight times that of general patients requiring airway management.

Anatomic and Physiological Changes during Pregnancy

Management of the patient's airway necessitates a thorough knowledge of the anatomic and physiological demands placed on the mother due to the growing fetus. Such changes have a tremendous impact on safe airway management of the patient.

Capillary engorgement of the mucosa throughout the respiratory tract causes swelling of the nasal and oral pharynx, larynx, and trachea. Elevated estrogen levels and increase in blood volume associated with pregnancy may also contribute to the mucosal edema. These changes may be markedly accentuated by a mild upper respiratory tract infection, fluid overload, preeclampsia, oxytocin infusion, or prolonged strenuous second stage of labor.

The progesterone-mediated smooth muscle relaxant effect on the gastrointestinal mucosa along with the anatomical changes secondary to the gravid uterus places the patient at risk for both regurgitation and pulmonary aspiration. Lower esophageal sphincter tone is decreased allowing gastric reflux and heart burn during pregnancy. Therefore, the patient is prone to silent regurgitation, active vomiting, and aspiration during impaired consciousness. Studies have shown that gastric emptying is slowed and mean gastric volume increases during labor. As the uterus enlarges, it impinges on the diaphragm, reducing the functional residual capacity. In addition, there is increased oxygen consumption and minute ventilation to meet the demands of the growing fetal-maternal unit. As a result, apnea in the pregnant patient results in a more rapid onset of hypoxia, hypercarbia, and acidosis than in nonpregnant patient. A patient may gain 10 kg or more during pregnancy. This weight gain results from the increased size of the uterus and fetus, increased volumes of blood and interstitial fluid, and deposition of fat. There is also a significant increase in breast size during pregnancy. Increased weight gain during pregnancy and large breast size can cause difficulty with intubation. Manipulation of the upper airway in a patient requires special attention. Placement of oral/nasal airways, suctioning, and careless laryngoscopy can result in airway trauma and bleeding. Manipulation of the nasal airway can lead to brisk epistaxis. Smaller size endotracheal tubes are recommended in patients due to the mucosal swelling, which also decreases the area of the glottic opening. Breast engorgement can hinder laryngoscopy, and so proper positioning is necessary along with the availability of a short-handled blade. Therefore positioning with blankets or use of a ramp under the shoulders can minimize the hazards of difficult laryngoscopy.

Airway Assessment

Most airway catastrophes occur when airway difficulty is not recognized prior to intubation. There are a few simple bedside tests that can be performed within a few seconds to evaluate the airway in a pregnant patient in the same manner as a nonpregnant patient. These tests include mouth opening, thyromental distance, Mallampati class, atlanto-occipital extension, and ability to protrude the mandible. No single test can reliably predict a difficult airway. A combination of these tests is essential to facilitate the management of the airway and to reduce the likelihood of adverse outcomes related to the airway. Predicting difficult airway enables the paramedic to implement appropriate care and thus avoid major airway catastrophes.

Preeclampsia and Airway-Related Changes

Preeclampsia is a multisystem disorder affecting approximately 8% of pregnancies. It is a pregnancy-associated disease occurring after 20-weeks' gestation and is characterized by hypertension, proteinuria, and edema. The cause still remains unknown but the understanding of pathophysiology has greatly increased. Women with preeclampsia have an increased risk of upper airway narrowing from pharyngolaryngeal edema. Reduced plasma proteins due to proteinuria and marked fluid retention, (especially in the head and neck region), increase the size of the tongue making it less mobile, causing more difficult identification of landmarks in preeclamptic patient's. In severe preeclampsia, edema of the face and neck should alert the paramedic to the possibility of difficult intubation, whereas edema of the tongue may herald imminent airway compromise. Preeclampsia accompanied by soft tissue edema and coagulopathy complicates repeated attempts at direct laryngoscopy causing laceration and bleeding in the upper airway. Marked upper airway edema and swelling of the tongue and soft tissues can be severe enough to cause total airway obstruction. Laryngeal edema can develop very rapidly in a preeclamptic patient without any warning signs such as facial edema, enlarged tongue, voice change or stridor; therefore, caution should be exercised. Dysphonia due to uvular edema has also been reported. Upper respiratory infection can further compromise the edematous airway in preeclampsia.

Morbid Obesity in Pregnancy and Airway

Morbid obesity in pregnancy is a growing problem and has a significant impact on maternal morbidity and mortality. It is associated with an increased risk for diabetes, hypertension, and preeclampsia. A recent study has shown that there is increased risk of postpartum hemorrhage, cesarean section for cephalo-pelvic disproportion, and gestational diabetes in morbidly obese patient when compared with nonobese patients. Obese women are at risk for airway complications, cardiopulmonary dysfunction, perioperative morbidity and mortality, and also pose technical challenges.

The airway of the obese patient can be very unpredictable. There is not only an increased risk of difficult intubation, but also increased difficulty in maintaining adequate mask ventilation in morbidly obese patients. In the supine position, breasts and chest wall soft tissue can hinder chest wall excursion and decrease compliance. Hood et al showed that difficult intubation was encountered more frequently in morbidly obese patient's (> 130 kg). Morbidly obese patients are at an increased risk of failed intubation and gastric aspiration during procedures requiring intubation.

Pregnancy is a state of high metabolic and physiological demand as mentioned earlier, but obese pregnant women are at double the risk for a difficult airway scenario.

Difficult Airway Management in Bariatric Patients

LEARNING OBJECTIVES

At the end of this chapter, you will be able to:

● Describe the key physiological changes that occur in obese patients.

● Identify the definitions for obesity as set forth by the World Health Organization.

● Review the strategies that can be used to minimize complications during intubation.

● Understand the technical difficulties that accompany airway management.

Introduction

Any patient can have a difficult airway, but obese patients have anatomic and physiological features that can make airway management particularly challenging. Obesity does not seem to be an independent risk factor for difficult intubation but is one of the several factors that need to be considered as part of an airway evaluation. To effectively manage airways in obese patients, health care providers working in the EMS setting must be proficient in airway evaluation and management in all types of patients.

Pulmonary Physiology

Obesity profoundly affects airway anatomy and pulmonary physiology. An understanding of these physiological changes, which may be exaggerated in the acutely ill patient, is necessary for proper airway management. The increased mortality in critically ill obese patients compared with nonobese patients can be attributed in part to the effect of obesity on the respiratory system. Diminished total lung capacity and vital capacity in obesity result from decreased chest wall compliance and increased abdominal cavity contents. Airway resistance is also increased in obesity. Obese individuals without significant obstructive lung disease or other underlying lung disease have a relatively high incidence of resting room air hypoxemia and hypercapnia, the cause of which is multifactorial. Diminished expiratory reserve volume results from collapse of the small airways; which results in decreased ventilation of the relatively well-perfused lung bases, causing ventilation-perfusion mismatch and hypoxemia. Ventilation-perfusion mismatching is exacerbated in the supine position and with sedation and paralysis, likely because of further alveolar collapse.

In addition, functional residual capacity declines exponentially as BMI increases, resulting in a smaller O_2 reserve and more rapid oxygen desaturation during periods of apnea. Obese individuals also have increased O_2 consumption and carbon dioxide production because of the metabolic activity of excess body tissue, and increased work of breathing.

Finally, obesity is associated with inefficient respiratory muscles, as evidenced by increased O_2 consumption during exercise compared with that of nonobese individuals. In addition to impaired pulmonary function, obese patients have alterations in gastrointestinal physiology that may affect airway management.

Bag-Valve-Mask Ventilation

Obese patients do not tolerate apnea well, and there may be time enough for only one attempt at tracheal intubation before critical oxygen desaturation. Thus, the ability to mask ventilate the obese patient is of utmost importance because paramedics traditionally rely on this rescue technique after failed attempts at tracheal intubation. Obesity has been demonstrated to predict difficult mask ventilation. A combination of poor chest wall compliance, decreased diaphragmatic excursion, increased upper airway resistance, and redundant supraglottic tissues makes mask ventilation more difficult in obese patients. Obesity as a predictor of difficult mask ventilation has not been studied in the ED setting, but one might anticipate obese patients to be even more difficult to adequately ventilate and oxygenate in cases of respiratory failure when lung compliance is often reduced. In situations in which mask ventilation is required, technique should be optimized with the use of oral or nasal airways, appropriately fitting mask, a two-person technique with a two-handed bilateral jaw thrust, and proper positioning of the patient in the ramped position.

Approach to Bariatric Airway Management

Preparation

Taking into consideration that unexpected difficulties may be encountered in the emergency setting, mask ventilation may be difficult or impossible, and the obese patient will rapidly undergo rapid O_2 desaturation during apneic periods, preparation, and careful planning are fundamental to the approaching the airway in obesity. The approach may vary considerably, depending on the clinical situation, operator experience, and resources available. The view below shows the different and effective devices and techniques in managing the airway in obesity. Once the decision is made to intubate, positioning the obese patient is arguably the most underappreciated technique in improving laryngoscopic view and ensuring successful tracheal intubation.

Positioning

Repositioning the morbidly obese patient after failed attempts can be difficult and time-consuming and proper positioning should be achieved before any attempts at laryngoscopy. In the morbidly obese patient, the head and shoulders should be elevated above the chest such that the external auditory canal is parallel with the sternal notch to optimize view during laryngoscopy. Multiple folded blankets placed under the head, shoulders, and neck may be required to achieve the so-called ramped position (Figure 11-9). The ramped position

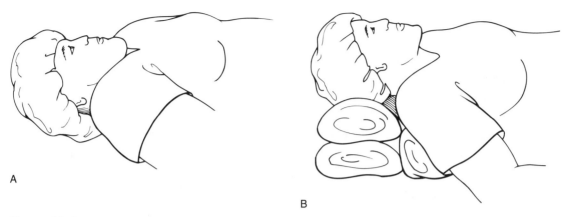

Figure 11-9 • Patient positioning.

improves laryngoscopic view over the standard "sniffing" position in obese patients. The ramped position may also improve mask ventilation and provide easy access to the neck for application of cricoid pressure and attempts at surgical airways. While properly positioning and preoxygenating the obese patient, the emergency physician must simultaneously decide the best approach to securing the airway.

Post-Tracheal Intubation Management

Confirmation

Reliance on indirect clinical tests alone, such as chest and gastric auscultation, chest excursions, endotracheal tube condensation, and O_2 saturations, to detect esophageal tracheal intubation contributes to hypoxemia, regurgitation, aspiration, and cardiovascular complications during emergency airway management. Obesity may further diminish the utility of clinical findings to confirm endotracheal tube placement.

Auscultation can be challenging because of excess chest wall tissue and pulse oximetry may be inaccurate because of poor lightwave transmission through increased soft tissue in the fingers. The use of devices such as capnography, disposable carbon dioxide detectors, and esophageal detectors has been advocated during emergency airway management to hasten the detection of and reduce the complications associated with esophageal tracheal intubation. However, esophageal detector devices may be less effective in morbidly obese patients. Interpretation of chest radiography can prove challenging as well, owing to poor penetration of radiographs through excess soft tissue. After confirmation of endotracheal tube placement, the clinician must next consider safe and effective mechanical ventilation techniques for obese patients.

Airway management in obese patients can be challenging because of the anatomic and physiological changes associated with this condition. Several techniques may help optimize airway management of the obese patient, including the use of CPAP during preoxygenation, proper positioning in the "ramped" position, and dosing of succinylcholine according to total bodyweight. The indications for tracheal intubation, the skills and experience of the operator, and the resources available will often dictate the technique used to secure the airway. When circumstances permit, consideration should be given to an awake approach to tracheal intubation in obese patients because facemask ventilation may be exceedingly difficult and O_2 desaturation may occur precipitously after the ablation of spontaneous ventilation.

Managing the Difficult Airway in Geriatric Patients

LEARNING OBJECTIVES

At the end of this chapter, you will be able to:

● Discuss the expected physiological changes that occur during the aging process.

● Identify related problems experienced by the geriatric patient airway management.

Introduction

US Census data estimate that 77 million Americans, or nearly 20% of the overall population, will be over age 65 by the year 2030. Similar trends are apparent throughout the developed world. The increase in the number of older adults has been accompanied by an increase in the use of health care, including the emergency department (ED), by patients with significant comorbid conditions such as diabetes, coronary artery disease (CAD), chronic obstructive pulmonary disease (COPD), and cancer.

Many older patients with comorbid disease will require airway management during the course of their illness. Increased patient age and its associated comorbidities affect airway management in three principal areas:

- Increased likelihood of requiring intubation during acute illness
- Increased difficulty performing bag-mask ventilation and intubation
- Adjustments in drug selection and dosing for rapid sequence intubation (RSI)

Geriatric Patient Airway Management

General overview:

- Advanced age can impact critical airway decision-making in three areas:
  - Elderly patients have diminished respiratory reserves.
  - Elderly patients have a high incidence of difficult airway resulting from poor mouth opening, missing teeth, and reduced cervical range of motion.
  - Ethical considerations.

Clinical considerations:

- Hypoxic elderly patients desaturate quickly, therefore earlier intubation of these patients should be considered.
- Remember to consider use of alternative devices such as CPAP.

Tips and techniques:

- Two-person BVM ventilation may be required due to difficulties getting mask seals.
- Reduced lung compliance and chest wall stiffness may make BVM ventilation difficult.
- Well-fitting dentures should be left in place during BVM ventilation and then removed for intubation.
- Etomidate is the preferred sedation agent in older patients because of its hemodynamic stability.

Cricothyroidotomy Surgical Airway

LEARNING OBJECTIVES

At the end of this chapter, you will be able to:

- Identify important anatomical landmarks for an emergency cricothyroidotomy.
- Identify the indications for performing an emergency cricothyroidotomy.
- Identify the proper equipment for performing an emergency cricothyroidotomy.
- Identify the procedural sequence for emergency cricothyroidotomy.
- Identify potential complications of emergency cricothyroidotomy.

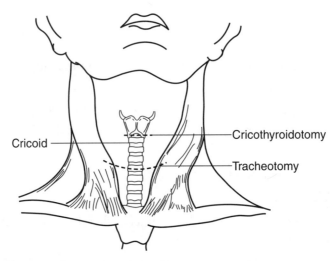

Figure 11-10 • Landmarks.
Reproduced with permission from Lalwani AK, ed. *CURRENT Diagnosis & Treatment in Otolaryngology—Head & Neck Surgery*. 3rd ed. 2012. New York: Copyright © McGraw-Hill Education. All rights reserved. Figure 38-4

Introduction

Indications

There are many reasons an emergency cricothyroidotomy may be required. Listed below are a few of the most common reasons:

- Obstructed airway: obstructed airway and/or swelling of tissues will usually prevent the passage of an ET through the airway. Therefore, a surgical airway distal to the obstruction is required. Causes of an obstructed airway include:
  - facial and oropharyngeal edema from burns
  - foreign objects (food or teeth)
- Congenital deformities of the oropharynx or nasopharynx will inhibit or prevent nasotracheal or orotracheal intubation.
- Trauma to the head and neck would preclude the use of an ambu-bag, oropharyngeal airway, nasopharyngeal airway and ET insertion. Examples include:
  - facial and oropharyngeal edema from severe trauma
  - facial fractures (mandible fracture)
  - nasal bone fractures
  - cribriform fractures

- Cervical spine fractures in a patient who needs an airway but whose intubation is unsuccessful or contraindicated.
- Last resort: health care provider is unable to establish an airway by any other means.

Cricothyroidotomy is a procedure in which the paramedic inserts a tracheostomy tube or modified ET through an incision in the cricothyroid membrane to establish an airway for oxygenation and ventilation. Cricothyroidotomy is indicated when an emergency airway is required and orotracheal or nasotracheal intubation is either unsuccessful or contraindicated. When the paramedic "cannot intubate and cannot ventilate" the patient, the swift establishment of an airway is crucial. Failure to provide oxygen to the brain within 3 to 5 minutes leads to anoxic encephalopathy and ultimately death. In a "cannot intubate and cannot ventilate" scenario, placement of an extraglottic airway device (ie, laryngeal mask airway) may be attempted as a rescue maneuver while preparation is made to perform a cricothyroidotomy. If oxygenation cannot be maintained, however, cricothyroidotomy is required.

Absolute contraindications: surgical cricothyroidotomy is absolutely contraindicated when the patient can be safely intubated either orally or nasally. Other absolute contraindications include complete transection of the trachea, laryngotracheal disruption with retraction of the distal trachea into the mediastinum, and fractured larynx.

Relative contraindications: surgical cricothyroidotomy is relatively contraindicated in young children for several reasons. The airway of a child is funnel-shaped, with the narrowest part located at the cricoid ring rather than at the vocal cords. This narrowing increases the risk for developing subglottic stenosis following cricothyroidotomy.

Procedure

- Palpate the landmarks (see Figure 11-11).
- Stabilize upper airway with nondominant hand is single most important factor in successful outcome.
- Perform midline vertical skin incision (see Figure 11-12).
- Palpate membrane through incision and enter with a horizontal incision at lower edge of membrane (see Figure 11-13).
- Dilate with a hemostat or Kelly clamp (see Figure 11-14).
- Place small (5.0) ET or tracheostomy tube (see Figure 11-15).

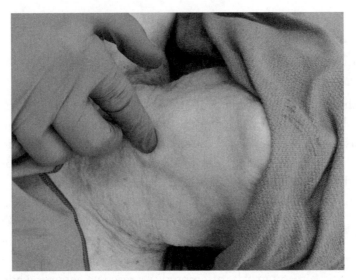

Figure 11-11 • Surgical airway landmark.
Reproduced with permission from Tintinalli JE, Stapczynski JS, Cline DM, Ma OJ, Cydulka RK, Meckler GD, eds. *Tintinalli's Emergency Medicine: A Comprehensive Study Guide.* 7th ed. 2011. New York: Copyright © McGraw-Hill Education. All rights reserved.

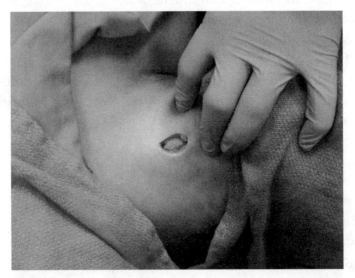

Figure 11-12 • Vertical skin incision.
Reproduced with permission from Tintinalli JE, Stapczynski JS, Cline DM, Ma OJ, Cydulka RK, Meckler GD, eds. *Tintinalli's Emergency Medicine: A Comprehensive Study Guide.* 7th ed. 2011. New York: Copyright © McGraw-Hill Education. All rights reserved.

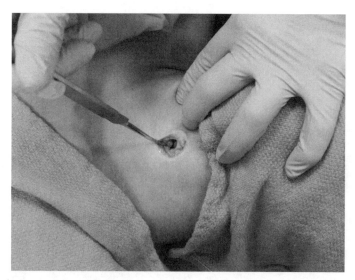

Figure 11-13 • Horizontal incision.
Reproduced with permission from Tintinalli JE, Stapczynski JS, Cline DM, Ma OJ, Cydulka RK, Meckler GD, eds. *Tintinalli's Emergency Medicine: A Comprehensive Study Guide.* 7th ed. 2011. New York:

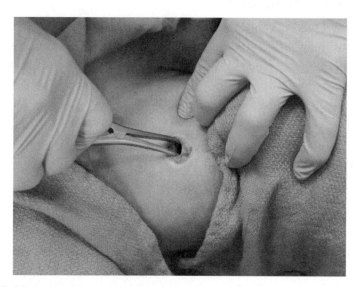

Figure 11-14 • Dilation with Kelly clamp.
Reproduced with permission from Tintinalli JE, Stapczynski JS, Cline DM, Ma OJ, Cydulka RK, Meckler GD, eds. *Tintinalli's Emergency Medicine: A Comprehensive Study Guide.* 7th ed. 2011. New York:

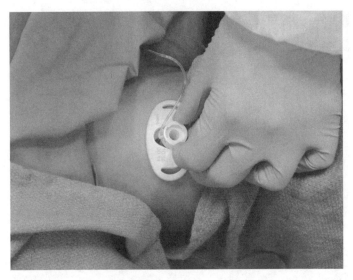

Figure 11-15 • Insertion of a tracheostomy tube.

Needle Cricothyroidotomy

When the paramedic "cannot intubate and cannot ventilate" the patient, the swift establishment of an airway is crucial. Failure to provide O_2 to the brain within 3 to 5 minutes leads to anoxic encephalopathy and ultimately death. Another means of getting O_2 to a patient with a compromised airway is to perform a needle cricothyroidotomy. This is performed by doing the following procedure:

1. Assemble equipment: 12 gauge Angiocath, 3 cc syringe, 3.0 ETT adapter, oxygen, BVM.

2. Place the patient in a supine position with support under the shoulders and mild hyperextension of the neck unless C-spine injury is suspected.

3. Palpate the neck in the midline and locate the slight depression just below the notch of the thyroid cartilage. This is the position of the cricothyroid membrane.

4. Prepare the area with Betadine® wipes.

5. Stabilize the airway between thumb and forefingers.

6. Insert the needle with catheter into the cricothyroid membrane at a 30-degree angle toward the patient's feet.

7. When the needle is through the membrane, stop and aspirate for air to ensure tracheal entry.

8. Advance the catheter over the needle and then remove the needle.

9. Attach the 3.0 ETT adapter to the hub of the catheter and begin ventilations with the BVM. Attach $EtCO_2$ monitor.

10. Secure the cannula with tape after confirming correct placement by auscultating for breath sounds (5 point check). Observe for kinking of cannula.

REVIEW QUESTIONS

1. Which of the following statements regarding the pediatric airway as compared with the adult airway is true?

    A. A child has a smaller tongue relative to the size of the oral cavity.
    B. An infant's epiglottis is relatively short and thicker.
    C. The vocal cords in infants have a higher attachment.
    D. In children younger than 10 years, the narrowest portion of the airway is below the vocal cords.

Correct answer is d.

2. A 4-month-old previously healthy male infant presents to EMS with cough and dyspnea for 2 days and a temperature of 38.4°C (101.1°F). There is no family history of asthma. He is tachypneic (respiratory rate, 48 breaths per minute) and has bilateral expiratory wheezing and subcostal retractions. His O_2 saturation is 93%. Which of the following is the most common cause of his illness?

    A. RSV
    B. Adenovirus
    C. Parainfluenza virus
    D. Mycoplasmal pneumonia

Correct answer is a.

3. Factors that predict difficult intubation in an obese patient include:

    A. short neck.
    B. thick neck.
    C. diabetes mellitus.
    D. abnormal upper teeth.
    E. All of the above.

Correct answer is e.

4. Obesity profoundly affects airway anatomy and pulmonary physiology.

    A. True.

    B. False.

Correct answer is a.

5. _____ _____ _____declines exponentially as BMI increases, resulting in a smaller O_2 reserve, and more rapid oxygen desaturation during periods of apnea.

    A. Reserve volume

    B. Functional residual capacity

    C. Work of breathing

    D. None of the above

Correct answer is b.

6. Obese individuals without significant obstructive lung disease or other underlying lung disease have a relatively high incidence of resting room air hypoxemia and hypercapnia.

    A. True.

    B. False.

Correct answer is a.

7. The first priority of trauma management and resuscitation is:

    A. head to toe survey.

    B. rapid completion of primary patient survey.

    C. ensuring a patent airway.

    D. control of external hemorrhage.

Correct answer is c.

8. A patient with a suspected flail chest develops increasing respirations and difficulty breathing. Which of the following interventions would be most likely to help the patient?

    A. Needle decompression

    B. Pericardiocentesis

    C. Administration of an analgesic

    D. Endotracheal intubation

Correct answer is d.

9. **The most common cause of airway obstruction in the unconscious patient is:**

   A. food bolus in the posterior pharynx.
   B. loss of tone in the submandibular muscles resulting in prolapse of the tongue into the posterior pharynx.
   C. collapse of the trachea due to loss of tone in the supporting muscles.
   D. laryngospasm owing to aspiration of oral secretions.

Correct answer is b.

10. **The jaw thrust maneuver for opening the airway has the advantage of the head tilt-chin lift maneuver in that:**

   A. it is easier to perform.
   B. it permits the use of either an oropharyngeal or nasopharyngeal airway.
   C. it can be performed without neck manipulation.
   D. it more closely approximates the natural airway anatomy.

Correct answer is c.

11. **Airway and respiratory care are paramount and early endotracheal intubation should be considered if patients present with symptoms of respiratory obstruction:**

   A. restlessness.
   B. air hunger.
   C. inability to swallow or drooling.
   D. a and b are correct.
   E. All of the above.

Correct answer is e.

12. **Prophylactic intubation is preferred in as controlled a fashion as possible rather than emergency intubation, cricothyroidotomy or tracheostomy.**

   A. True.
   B. False.

Correct answer is a.

13. The presence of a bleeding neck wound shouldn't detract from an airway injury, respiratory distress, stridor, and altered level of consciousness mandating emergency airway management. The importance of this process cannot be emphasized too much; approximately 90% of patients with penetrating neck injuries present with airway compromise.

    A. True.
    B. False.

Correct answer is b. Approximately 10% of patients with penetrating neck injuries present with airway compromise.

14. Surgical cricothyroidotomy is absolutely contraindicated when the patient can be safely intubated either orally or nasally. Other absolute contraindications include complete transection of the trachea, laryngotracheal disruption with retraction of the distal trachea into the mediastinum, and fractured larynx.

    A. True.
    B. False.

Correct answer is a.

15. Advanced age can impact critical airway decision-making in three areas:

    A. Elderly patients have diminished respiratory reserves.
    B. Elderly patients have a high incidence of difficult airway resulting from poor mouth opening, missing teeth and reduced cervical range of motion.
    C. Ethical considerations.
    D. All the above are correct.

Correct answer is d.

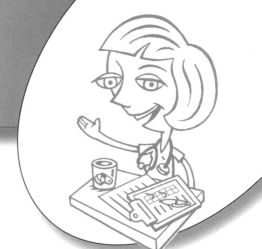

chapter **12**

Continuous Positive Airway Pressure (CPAP)

LEARNING OBJECTIVES

At the end of this chapter, you will be able to:

① Record three negative physiologic effects of acute pulmonary edema.

② Present three focused history questions a provider might use to effectively identify acute pulmonary edema.

③ Define the letters in the pneumonic CPAP.

④ Define PEEP.

⑤ List at least three positive physiologic effects of CPAP.

⑥ Record at least two specific, therapeutic benefits of CPAP for the acute pulmonary edema patient.

⑦ List at least four precautions for the use of CPAP.

⑧ List at least four components of the exclusion criteria for the use of CPAP.

> ## KEY TERMS
>
> | | |
> |---|---|
> | Calcium antagonist overdose | Non-cardiogenic pulmonary edema |
> | CPAP | Pulmonary edema |
> | High altitude pulmonary edema | Salicylate overdose |

Scenario

You are called to a doctor's clinic on Main Street. As you arrive, you met at the front door by one of the nurses who states Dr. Mike is in treatment room 1 treating a 65-year-old man with a history of alcohol abuse who came in with shortness of breath. His symptoms have been present for the past 1 day. He has a cough, productive with blood tinged sputum and chest pain. His vital signs include: BP 180/94, P 110, RR 28, T 98.9, and $SpO_2 = 90\%$ on 4L nasal cannula. His pulmonary examination includes rales on the left and right lower lung fields.

What is your diagnosis? And how would you begin treating him?

Introduction

Pulmonary edema is one of the most serious and life-threatening situations an EMT and paramedic responds to. Lately, it has become apparent that in most cases, pulmonary edema is not caused by fluid accumulation, but rather fluid redistribution that is directed into the lungs because of heart failure. Pulmonary edema is a combination of marked increase in systemic vascular resistance superimposed on insufficient systolic and diastolic myocardial functional reserve. This resistance results in increased left ventricular diastolic pressure causing increased pulmonary venous pressure, which yields a fluid shift from the intravascular compartment into the pulmonary interstitium and alveoli, inducing pulmonary edema. Therefore, the emphasis in treating pulmonary edema has shifted from diuretics (ie, furosemide) to vasodilators (ie, high-dose nitrates) combinedwith noninvasive positive airway pressure ventilation. This chapter will explore the pathogenesis of pulmonary edema and the evolving management strategies.

Pathophysiology of Pulmonary Edema

The lymphatic system can remove an estimated 10 to 20 mL of fluid per hour in the normal, healthy lung. Under stress, the lymphatic system can remove additional fluid through increased flow. When this capability is exceeded, fluid initially accumulates in the interstitial spaces, resulting in interstitial edema. When the volume exceeds the capacity of the interstitium, the tight junctions of the alveolar epithelium are damaged, and the fluid floods into the alveolar air spaces.

It's generally accepted that two mechanisms are primarily responsible for pulmonary edema. The first is excessive pressure within the pulmonary circulation, which increases the hydrostatic pressure within the peri-alveolar microvasculature and the rate of fluid transfer into the interstitial space. Although many potential cardiac and noncardiac causes exist, among the most common cardiac causes are increasing pressure within the left atrium secondary to left ventricular failure, valvular heart disease (VHD), and hypertension. When this fluid enters the interstitial spaces lung compliance decreases, and airway resistance increases. Additionally, fluid in the alveoli decreases the surface area available for gas exchange and alters lung capacity. These changes aren't uniform, resulting in an alteration of lung ventilation.

The second primary mechanism is increased permeability of the microvasculature. The list of diseases that can cause increased permeability is lengthy and includes pulmonary contusions, aspiration, carbon monoxide poisoning, aspirin overdoses, near-drowning, narcotic overdose, high altitude, and chemical inhalation pneumonias.

The mechanisms by which these conditions result in pulmonary edema vary widely. For example, shock and hypoxemia resulting from narcotic overdoses can cause alveolar capillary damage. Excessive infusion of fluids by prehospital personnel makes the condition worse.

As stated earlier, pulmonary edema develops when the movement of fluid from the blood vessels to the interstitial space and in some instances to the alveoli exceeds the return of fluid to the blood by way of the lymphatics. Whether initiated by an imbalance of Starling forces or by primary damage to the various components of the alveolar capillary membrane, the sequence of fluid exchange and gathering in the lungs is the same and can be represented as three separate stages.

In stage 1, there is an increase in transfer of liquid from blood capillaries to the interstitial space. The pulmonary capillary endothelial junctions are widened by an increase in filtrative forces or by toxic damage of the membrane. Despite the increased filtration, there is no increase in interstitial volume because there is an equal increase in lymphatic drainage. When the filtered load from the pulmonary capillaries to the interstitial space is increased beyond a limit, the lymphatics cannot follow this rapid rhythm and liquid and colloid begin to accumulate in the more compliant interstitial compartment surrounding bronchioles, arterioles and venules (stage 2). With further increase in filtered load, the volume limits of the more compliant spaces of the interstitial space are exceeded and the liquid begins to accumulate in the less compliant compartments of the interstitial space. The alveolar capillary membrane is very thin and disrupts immediately, so that alveolar flooding occurs (stage 3). This flooding decreases pulmonary oxygenation which results in deterioration of left ventricular function. This mechanism leads to further increase of pressure in the pulmonary capillaries and further deterioration of pulmonary edema.

Non-cardiogenic Causes of Pulmonary Edema

- Narcotic overdose
- Salicylate intoxication
- Calcium antagonist overdose
- High altitude

Narcotic Overdose

Pulmonary edema is usually a complication of pharmaceutical intoxication with antidepressants or opiates. It is a well-recognized complication of heroin overdose and represents the most important cardiopulmonary toxic effect of opiate overdosing.

It is usually a standard pathologic finding in fatal cases and may be the result of intravenous, oral or administration of the narcotic drug by inhalation. The pathophysiologic feature of the syndrome is increased permeability of pulmonary capillaries and the normal or even low left atrial pressure. The mechanisms which are responsible for the endothelial damage remain unclear.

In spite of the fact that pulmonary edema usually appears shortly after heroin injection, it may appear late, even 6 hours later. Mechanical ventilation with positive end-expiratory pressure (PEEP) offers great support to patients.

Salicylate Intoxication

Salicylate intoxication is frequently overlooked as a cause of noncardiogenic pulmonary edema and altered mental status in adult patients. Non-early diagnosis and treatment leads to high morbidity and mortality. A high index of suspicion is necessary for early recognition and successful treatment with hemodialysis and urinary alkalization.

Calcium Antagonist Overdose

Noncardiogenic pulmonary edema has been reported after an overdose of diltiazem, nifedipine, and verapamil. Multiple cellular mechanisms appear to be responsible for the development of noncardiogenic pulmonary edema after overdoses of calcium channel blockers. First, prostaglandins have been shown to play an important role in maintaining cellular integrity, especially during lung inflation.

The protective role of prostaglandins in cellular integrity is lost with excessive concentrations of calcium channel blockers (inhibition of prostacyclin release). This leads to a "leaky capillary syndrome." Secondly, calcium channel blockers, cause systemic pre-capillary vasodilation and peripheral edema due to their effect on vascular smooth muscle. Finally, it has been shown that the pulmonary vasodilatory effect of calcium antagonists may lead to perfusion ventilation mismatch and hypoxemia. Management of these patients includes infusion of calcium and catecholamines and correction of hyperglycemia.

High-Altitude

This uncommon type of non-cardiogenic pulmonary edema occurs in young people who have quickly ascended to altitudes above 8825 ft (2700 m) and who then engage in strenuous physical exercise at that altitude, before they have become acclimatized. The incidence of this illness is about 6.5 cases per 100 exposures in persons less than 21 years of age. Although most patients have pulmonary hypertension, the pulmonary capillary wedge pressure is normal. The direct effect of alveolar hypoxia on increasing alveolar-capillary membrane permeability is considered possible mechanism for the pathogenesis of noncardiogenic pulmonary edema. Transient intravascular coagulation has also been implicated. Gradual ascent, allowing time for acclimatization and limiting physical exertion for 2 to 3 days in high altitudes are thought to be preventive. Reversal of this syndrome is rapid (in less than 48 hours) and certain by returning the patient to alower altitude and by administering a high inspiratory concentration of oxygen. When this is not available, treatment with nifedipine is recommended until descent is possible.

In near-drowning cases, aspirated water and subsequent loss of surfactant, as well as other factors, contribute to pulmonary edema. In severe cases of CO poisoning, pulmonary edema may result from a cascade of events surrounding free radical production and cellular damage. High-altitude pulmonary edema (HAPE) occurs when an individual ascends to high altitudes and remains there for 24 to 48 hours or longer. Our discussion will primarily focus on the first mechanism of pulmonary edema described—excessive pressure within the pulmonary circulation. Heart failure can be subdivided into left- and right-sided heart failure. Right-sided heart failure refers to an increase in intraventricular or intra-atrial pressure resulting from pump inefficiency that causes systemic venous congestion. Left-sided heart failure refers to symptoms associated with the increase of pressure within the left side of the heart, which is transmitted to the pulmonary circulation.

Additionally, heart failure can be further classified as being caused by impairment of contractility (ie, systolic dysfunction) or impairment of ventricular filling (ie, diastolic dysfunction). Either way, cardiac output suffers. Initially, cardiac output may be temporarily increased due to elevated heart rate and sympathetic tone. This results in higher cardiac oxygen demand, further injuring the heart. Eventually, the heart depletes its own catecholamine stores and becomes less responsive to further sympathetic stimulation. As the condition continues, ventricular remodeling takes place with myocardial hypertrophy and ventricular dilatation.

How Does CPAP Work?

Continous positive airway pressure is not a true ventilator because it does not actively assist inspiration. It requires a spontaneously breathing patient and is unable to support ventilation in the case of apnea. CPAP often is confused with PEEP. CPAP is a specific mode of mechanical ventilation, whereas PEEP is the elevation of baseline system pressure during other positive-pressure modes of ventilation.

Principles of Operation

By delivering a constant pressure during both inspiration and expiration, CPAP increases functional residual capacity opening collapsed or underventilated alveoli and improves oxygenation. The increase in functional residual capacity may also improve lung compliance, decreasing the work of breathing. In addition, application of CPAP in acute pulmonary edema lowers left ventricular trans-mural pressure, reducing in this way afterload and increases cardiac output. Further, by counterbalancing the inspiratory threshold load imposed by intrinsic positive end-expiratory pressure (PEEPi), CPAP may reduce the work of breathing in patients with COPD. In this case, portable Bi-level positive airway pressure (BiPAP) devices are used. These devices deliver a low CPAP in expiration (named expiratory positive airway pressure—EPAP) which cycles with a higher pressure which assists inspiration (inspiratory positive airway pressure—IPAP).

Continous positive airway pressure is employed in patients with acute respiratory failure to correct hypoxemia. Indications for the use of CPAP include the following:

1. Cardiogenic pulmonary edema

2. Patients with decompensated obstructive sleep apnea (when respiratory acidosis is present noninvasive ventilation in the form of bi-level pressure support should be used)

3. Patients with chest wall trauma, particularly those with multiple rib fractures and flail chest.

4. Diffuse pneumonia, especially in immune-compromised patients in whom invasive mechanical ventilation presents many complications.

5. Asthma and COPD

The only variables set by the paramedic are the level of CPAP and the sensitivity of the demand system (if it is included in the device). Pressures commonly used to deliver CPAP to patients with acute respiratory distress range from 5 to 12 cm H_2O. Typically, application of CPAP starts with low pressures, about 4 to 5 cm H_2O, and gradually pressure is titrated upward under close monitoring of SpO_2 and patient's respiratory rate. Optimum CPAP pressure is achieved when a maximum SpO_2 is reached, the respiratory rate is reduced and the delivered pressure is well tolerated by the patient with minimal leaks. In patients with acute respiratory distress and severe hypoxemia a higher CPAP pressure may be necessary from the beginning of application to stabilize gas exchange.

Contraindications for the Use of CPAP

- Patient less than 8 years of age
- Unable to maintain a patent airway
- Decreased level of consciousness (LOC)

- Pneumothorax
- Systolic BP < 90 mm Hg
- Recent surgery to face or mouth
- Epistaxis
- Patient unable to tolerate mask or pressure

What Went Wrong?

Continous positive airway pressure splints the alveoli open, thereby preventing alveolar collapse and allowing unimpeded alveolar ventilation. CPAP also decreases preload and afterload, improves lung compliance, increases functional residual capacity, and decreases work of breathing. The use of CPAP also decreases hospital stays. The typical level of pressure provided by CPAP in acute cardiogenic pulmonary edema is 5 to 10 cm of water. CPAP requires a high gas flow to achieve this pressure. Pressure within the circuit is held constant regardless of flow by use of threshold resistors, which open to allow expiration when pressure is excessive. This valve is often a simple spring device.

REVIEW QUESTIONS

1. **Which of the following is the primary pulmonary abnormality involved in congestive heart failure?**

   A. Loss of elasticity of the alveoli
   B. Bronchospasm of the terminal bronchioles
   C. Fluid collection in the alveoli
   D. Poor perfusion of the lung

   Correct answer is c.

2. **Which of the following patients may benefit from the application of CPAP?**

    A. 67-year-old woman who suddenly became short of breath while walking to get a glass of water in the middle of the night. She is overweight, sleeps propped up on a number of pillows, has a history of MI, NIDDM, and CHF. Vitals: HR 112, RR 36, BP 180/98, SpO$_2$ 93%, showing signs of accessory muscle use. Auscultation: crackles in the bases.

    B. 28-year-old woman who is short of breath after walking outside on a very cold winter day. She has a history of asthma but forgot her inhaler at home. Vitals: HR 102, RR 36, BP 146/96, SpO$_2$ 96%, auscultation: expiratory wheezing throughout.

    C. 59-year-old man complaining of localized chest pain and shortness of breath. He claims he saw his family doctor today who gave him an antibiotic. Vitals: HR 90, RR 26, BP 150/90, SpO$_2$ 96%, auscultation: crackles mid-left lobe.

    D. 14-year-old adolescent who was playing soccer and can't seem to catch her breath. Her mother states she has been undergoing tests for asthma but nothing is yet confirmed. HR 120, RR 36, BP 130/86, SpO$_2$ 97%, auscultation: wheezing throughout.

Correct answer is a.

3. **CPAP works primarily by which of the following mechanisms?**

    A. Reversing bronchospasm
    B. "Splinting" the lung by keeping the alveoli expanded
    C. Forcing oxygen into the blood stream
    D. Maintaining an open airway

Correct answer is b.

4. **As ventilation worsens, which of the following describes the differences in oxygen and carbon dioxide concentrations?**

    A. Oxygen saturation and carbon dioxide concentrations go up.
    B. Carbon dioxide concentration and oxygen saturation go down.
    C. Oxygen saturation goes up and carbon dioxide concentration gradually goes down.
    D. Carbon dioxide concentration goes up and oxygen saturation gradually goes down.

Correct answer is d.

5. **Which of the following is the primary pulmonary abnormality involved in emphysema?**

    A. Bronchospasm of the terminal bronchioles
    B. Fluid collection in the alveoli
    C. Loss of elasticity of the alveoli
    D. Poor perfusion of the lung

Correct answer is c.

6. Which of the following is a potential complication associated with the treatment of asthma using CPAP?

   A. Increased gas exchange due to splinting of the alveoli.
   B. Alveolar collapse leading to decreased surface area for gas exchange.
   C. Increased mucous production.
   D. Increased air trapping and intrathoracic pressure.

Correct answer is d.

7. Which of the following represents the potential assessment findings of a patient with pneumonia?

   A. Patient complains of shortness of breath, refuses to lay down on your stretcher, and auscultation reveals crackles in both bases and mid-lobes.
   B. Patient complains of shortness of breath, localized chest pain, pain on inspiration, and a productive cough; auscultation reveals crackles in the right lower lobe (near the pain).
   C. Patient complains of acute onset shortness of breath while bringing in the groceries from the car, she has tried to use her inhaler but it isn't working. Auscultation reveals wheezing in all fields.
   D. Patient complains of shortness of breath and localized chest pain. Incident history reveals signs and symptoms began immediately after sneezing. Auscultation reveals absent air entry to the left lower lobe (near the pain).

Correct answer is b.

8. Which of the following indicates the primary reason for application of CPAP to patients in severe respiratory distress?

   A. Patients who receive CPAP treatment in the prehospital setting are less likely to require intubation.
   B. CPAP enables the paramedic to deliver a higher amount of oxygen in a shorter amount of time to patients needing high concentration oxygen.
   C. The use of CPAP enables the paramedic to be hands free as opposed to using a BVM for those patients to require assisted ventilations.
   D. CPAP treatment is faster and more effective than BVM ventilation for patients with CHF.

Correct answer is a.

9. Which of the following indicates the correct path of air through the respiratory system?

   A. Nose, larynx, pharynx, trachea, bronchi, bronchioles, alveoli
   B. Nose, pharynx, larynx, trachea, bronchioles, bronchi, alveoli
   C. Nose, larynx, pharynx, trachea, bronchioles, bronchi, alveoli
   D. Nose, pharynx, larynx, trachea, bronchi, bronchioles, alveoli

Correct answer is d.

10. **Which of the following causes of shortness of breath would occur due to a decrease in perfusion?**

    A. Pulmonary embolism

    B. Asthma attack

    C. Pneumonia

    D. Pulmonary edema

Correct answer is a.

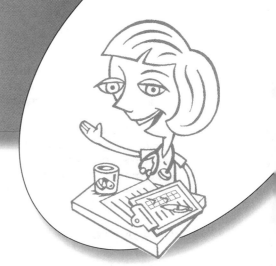

Key Terms

ABG: Arterial blood gas, a test that analyzes arterial blood for oxygen (O_2), carbon dioxide (CO_2) and bicarbonate content in addition to blood pH. This test is used to test the effectiveness of ventilation.

Acidosis: a pathologic state characterized by an increase in the concentration of hydrogen ions in the arterial blood above the normal level. May be caused by an accumulation of CO_2 or acidic products of metabolism or by a decrease in the concentration of alkaline compounds.

Acinus: also called the primary lobule, and is the functioning end of the airway where gas exchange takes place; includes the alveoli, respiratory bronchioles, and alveolar ducts.

Alkalosis: a state characterized by a decrease in the hydrogen ion concentration of arterial blood below normal level. The condition may be caused by an increase in the concentration of alkaline compounds, or by decrease in the concentration of acidic compounds or CO_2.

Alveolar macrophages: type 3 phagocytic scavenger cells in the lung.

Alveolar–capillary membrane: This is the barrier to diffusion from the air in the alveoli to the hemoglobin contained in the red blood cells (RBCs).

Angle of Louis: the slight defection between the body of the sternum and the manubrium at the level of the second rib just in front of the carina.

Anoxia: this can be the result of poor supply or absence of oxygen to the lungs. It can also occur when the blood is not able to carry O_2 to the tissue or when the tissues are unable to absorb the oxygen from the blood.

Anterior and posterior nares: the end of the nostrils which open into the nasal space, that allow breathing in and out in the nose. Each nare is an oval opening measuring about 1.5 cm in length and about 1 cm across. Posterior nares are a pair of openings in the back of the nasal cavity. They connect the nasal cavity with the upper throat and allow the flow of air.

Apices of lungs: the narrow superior portion of the lung that protrude 2-3 cm above the clavicle.

Asphyxia: absence of O_2 and accumulation of CO_2.

Asthma: a condition, often of allergic origin, that is marked by labored breathing with wheezing and a feeling of tightness in the chest. It is caused by the contracting of smooth muscle around the airways known as bronchospasm which constricts the airways making it difficult to breathe.

Atelectasis: a collapse of lung tissue preventing the exchange of O_2 and CO_2.

Bronchi: the airways which lead into the lungs and eventually the alveoli. They consist of the main-stem, lobar, segmental, sub-segmental bronchi and eventually bronchioles.

Bronchioles: within the broncho-pulmonary segments ultimately branch into terminal bronchioles.

Bronchodilation: an enlargement of the respiratory passageways caused by relaxing the smooth muscles around the airway.

Capnogram: the wave form.

Capnography: the measurement of CO_2 in exhaled breath.

Capnometer: numeric measurement of CO_2

Carbon dioxide (CO_2): a byproduct of cellular metabolism that is exhaled during the respiratory cycle.

Carboxyhemoglobin: formed when CO_2 binds with hemoglobin. It is one of the ways that CO_2 is transported through the blood system from the cells to the lungs.

Carina: The carina is where the trachea splits (bifurcates) into the right and left main-stem bronchi.

Chronic obstruction pulmonary disease (COPD): a disease process involving chronic inflammation of the airways, including chronic bronchitis (disease in the large airways) and emphysema (disease located in smaller airways and alveolar regions). The obstruction is generally permanent and progressive over time.

Cricoid cartilage: a ring-shaped cartilage, which forms the inferior margin of the trachea. It is the only circular ring of cartilage of the larynx.

Dead space: areas within the respiratory system that do not participate in gas exchange. These areas can be anatomical, alveolar, or mechanical.

Dead space ventilation: portions of the lung which normally partake in gas exchange, but because of lack of perfusion, are no longer able to do so.

Diamox ™: a carbonic anhydrase inhibitor that decreases H+ ion secretion and increases HCO3 excretions by the kidneys, causing a diuretic effect.

Diaphragm: a large respiratory muscle that separates the thoracic cavity from the abdominal-pelvic cavity. It is a very energy efficient muscle that rarely tires. (Only seen in chronic lung disease.)

Diffusion: is the movement of molecules from an area of high concentration to an area of low concentration. It is the guiding principle behind O_2 and CO_2 exchange. Gases move from the lungs to the blood stream because of the pressure difference (high to low) between the two areas.

Embolism: an air bubble or clot in the blood stream.

Emphysema: a disease of the alveoli which decreases the surface area where the lungs become floppy and collapse to trap air and the patient has a hard time expiring.

End tidal CO_2 (ETCO$_2$ or PetCO$_2$): level of partial pressure CO_2 released at the end of expiration.

Epiglottis: a spoon shaped flap of elastic cartilage to help guide food into the esophagus and keep it out of the airway.

Eustachian tubes: are connecting passageways that aid in equalizing middle ear pressure.

External obliques: are muscles that compress the abdomen and rotate the trunk laterally. Used during forced exhalation and exercising.

Fissures: separates the lobes of the lungs. There are two: horizontal and oblique.

Glottis: the opening through the vocal cord.

Goblet cells: found in the lamina propria which produces mucous.

Hering-Breuer inflation reflex: pulmonary stretch receptors that lie within the airway smooth muscle that respond to the distension of the lung. They respond reflexively by slowing the respiratory rate and preventing excessive lung inflation.

Hilum: the spot at which the main-stem bronchi enter each lung.

Hypercapnia: the presence of an excessive amount of CO_2 in the blood.

Hyperventilation: a state in which there is an increased amount of air entering the pulmonary alveoli (increased alveolar ventilation), resulting in reduction of carbon dioxide tension and eventually leading to alkalosis.

Hypopharynx: lies between the base of the tongue and the entrance to the esophagus.

Hypotension: the presence of abnormally low blood pressure.

Hypothermia: abnormally low body temperature.

Hypoventilation: a state in which there is a reduced amount of air entering the pulmonary alveoli.

Hypovolemia: diminished volume of circulating blood in the body.

Hypoxemia: low O_2 in the blood. Specifically, hypoxemia is determined by measuring the partial pressure of oxygen in the arterial blood (PaO_2).

Hypoxia: low O_2 in the body often specified, i.e. anemic hypoxia, hypoxic hypoxia, histotoxic hypoxia, and stagnant hypoxia.

Iatrogenic: any condition induced in a patient by the effects of medical treatment.

Inflation reflex (Hering-Breuer reflex): the reflex that prevents us from over inflating our lungs.

Intercostals: a muscle group on the chest wall between the ribs that aid in breathing.

Internal obliques: an accessory breathing muscle group in the abdomen.

Irritant receptors: sensors that detect chemicals in the nose to stimulate a sneeze.

Kussmaul's respirations: abnormal breathing pattern brought on by strenuous exercise or metabolic acidosis, and is characterized by an increased ventilatory rate, very large tidal volume, and no expiratory pause.

Lamina propria: a sub mucosal layer of the airway that contains tiny blood vessels, fibrous tissue, lymphatic vessels, sub mucosal glands and nerve fibers.

Lingua: the section of the left lung that is equal to the middle lobe on the right lung.

Lobes: the lungs are divided into sections that are called lobes. The right lung has three lobes, (superior, middle, inferior) and have two fissures, (horizontal, oblique) in the right lung that separates the lobes. The left lung has two lobes, (superior, inferior) and a single fissure, (oblique) that defines the two lobes.

Manubrium: part of the sternum it is the widest and most superior part. It articulates with clavicle and the cartilage of the first ribs.

Mast cells: are mobile connective tissue cells located near blood flow. In regards to the anatomy and physiology of the lungs, mast cells are located in the sub mucosal layer of the tracheobronchial tree. The mast cells act as messenger's cells and when irritated, during an allergic asthma attack, may release potent chemicals like histamine, heparin, leukotrienes, and prostaglandin. The histamine causes swelling and bronchospasms in the tracheobronchial tree.

Mediastinum: between the lungs, in a space called the mediastinum, lie the heart, the great vessels (the aorta and two-vena cava), the esophagus, the trachea, the major bronchi, and many nerves.

Mucosa: mucous membrane: similar to skin, in that the mucosa provides a protective barrier against bacterial invasion. Mucous membranes differ from skin in that they secrete mucus, a watery substance that lubricates the openings.

Nasopharynx: the upper part of the pharynx continuous with the nasal passages. The lining of the nasopharynx gives off watery secretions and helps to moisten the air as we breathe. Air enters through the mouth more rapidly and directly. As a result, it is less moist than air that enters through the nose.

Oropharynx: the part of the back of the throat that is behind the tongue. Conducts both food from the mouth and air from the nose.

Oxygen delivery system: a device used to deliver O_2 concentrations above ambient air to the lungs through the upper airway.

Oxygenation: the process of supplying, treating or mixing with O_2.

Oxyhemoglobin: hemoglobin in combination with O_2.

PaCO$_2$: the partial pressure of CO_2 in the blood.

Palate: the roof of the mouth; the front part being hard and bony and the back palate is soft and protects the nose from swallow liquids.

Parietal pleura: the outer lining of the lungs.

Pectoralis major: the 'pecs', the chest muscles of the upper thorax.

Pericardium: the sac-like outer lining of the heart.

Phrenic nerve: a nerve formed in the neck which innervates the diaphragm. It leaves the spinal column between C2 and C5, and bifurcates in the thoracic cavity. Each limb (2) of the split nerve has a corresponding 'hemi-diaphragm.'

Pleura: a thin layer of mesothelial tissue found in the thoracic cavity. The pleura cover the outside of the lungs. The visceral pleura are the inner layer covering the lungs and the outer layer, the parietal pleura, lines the inside of the thoracic cavity. The two pleura's adhere to each other due to the lubricating secretions which allow the pleura to glide over each other easily for friction free movement.

Pneumonia: a lung disease in which viral or bacterial caused inflammation causes an accumulation of fluid and cellular debris in the alveoli preventing gas exchange.

Pneumothorax: an abnormal state characterized by the presence of gas (as air) in the pleural cavity.

Pores of Kohn: small openings between alveoli, allowing air to move between individual air sacs. The number of pores increases with age.

Pulmonary embolism: the lodgment of a blood clot in the lumen of a pulmonary artery, causing a severe dysfunction in respiratory function.

Pulmonary surfactant: a chemical secreted in the lungs to keep the lungs open by reducing surface tension in the alveoli.

Rectus abdominus: the stomach muscles that make up the "six pack" in front of the abdomen.

Scalenes: neck muscles that help inspiratory effort, accessory muscles of breathing.

Septum: the middle partition separating the right and left nostrils.

Shunt perfusion: areas of the lungs that are perfused but not ventilated which leads to an absence of gas exchange.

Sternomastoids: accessory muscles that are prominent on the side of the neck.

Sternum: the flat bone in the center of the chest between the ribs.

Thyrotoxicosis: toxic condition due to hyperactivity of the thyroid gland. Symptoms include rapid heart rate, tremors, increased metabolic basal metabolism, nervous symptoms and loss of weight.

Trachea: the main breathing tube from the neck to the lungs.

Transverse abdominus: accessory breathing muscles.

Turbinates: three washboard bones that increase the surface area of the inner nose for greater humidification and cause turbulent flow pattern to mix the air so that foreign particles impact in mucosa.

V: Q Mismatch: an imbalance between ventilation compared to perfusion as occurs with shunt perfusion and dead space ventilation.

Ventilation/perfusion ratio (V/Q): the comparative ratio of air to blood in the lungs.

Vertebra: one of 24 bones making up the spine. The 12 thoracic vertebrae have ribs attached.

Visceral pleura: the inner lining of the two linings surrounding the lungs.

Xyphoid process: the dagger-like tip at the base of the sternum.

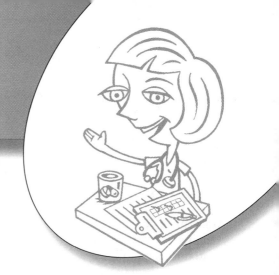

Index

Note: Page numbers followed by *f* or *t* indicate figures or tables, respectively.

A

ABG. *See* Arterial blood gas (ABG)
Acetylcholine
   metabolism of, 113–114
   as neurotransmitter, 180–181
Acetylcholinesterase inhibition, 114
Acetylcysteine, 119–120
Acid-base balance, 34–38
Acid-base disorders. *See* Acidosis;
     Alkalosis
Acidosis
   ABG values in, 43, 44–45
   compensation in, 46–47
   metabolic. *See* Metabolic acidosis
   respiratory. *See* Respiratory
     acidosis
Acute respiratory distress syndrome (ARDS),
    149, 158
Adventitia, 9
Aerosol mask, 102, 103*f*
Aerosol treatment, for cough, 119
Air
   alveolar, 96, 96*t*
   atmospheric, 94, 95, 96*t*
Airway management
   in burn patients, 262–265

cricothyroidectomy for.
    See Cricothyroidotomy
endotracheal intubation for. *See* Endotracheal
    intubation
in geriatric patients, 272–273
in head injured patients, 259–262
in obese patients. *See* Obese patients
in pediatric patients. *See* Pediatric
    patients
in pregnant patient. *See* Pregnant patients
simple artificial airways for, 202–203
simple maneuvers for, 201–202
suction for, 203
in trauma patients, 256–259
Albuterol
   for asthma, 123
   dosing in pediatric patients, 243
   mechanisms of action of, 111, 126
   pharmacology of, 126–127
Alkalosis
   ABG values in, 44, 45–46
   compensation in, 46–47
   metabolic. *See* Metabolic alkalosis
   respiratory. *See* Respiratory alkalosis
Alpha-1-antitrypsin deficiency, 125
Alpha$_1$-agonists, 114–115
Alpha$_2$-agonists, 115–116

Alveolar-arterial gradient, 76
Alveolar-capillary (respiratory) membrane, 15–16, 75f
Alveolar cells, 13, 14f
Alveolar macrophage, 15
Alveolus
  anatomy of, 13, 14f
  gas exchange in, 96
  partial pressures in, 95–96, 96t
Aminophylline, 127
Anaphylactic reaction, 130
Anatomic shunt, 67
Anatomical dead space, 19
Anemic hypoxia, 64, 64t
Anti-tussives, 117
Aortic regurgitation, 147
Aortic stenosis, 147
Apert syndrome, 246–247
Apnea, 143t
Apneustic area, 26
Apneustic breathing, 143t
ARDS (acute respiratory distress syndrome), 149, 158
Arrhythmias, pulse oximetry in, 87
Arterial blood gas (ABG)
  in acid-base imbalances, 42–46
  for blood oxygen evaluation, 52
  components of, 41
  key points, 42
Aspiration pneumonia, 151
Asthma
  exacerbation, capnography during, 79, 82f
  pathogenesis of, 121, 144, 241
  in pediatric patients, 241–243
  physiology of, 120–121
  treatment of, 122–124, 144. See also Continuous positive airway pressure (CPAP)
Ataxic respirations, 143t
Atrial myxoma, 147
Atropine
  in pediatric patients, 251
  in rapid sequence intubation, 171–172, 178, 259
Auscultation sites, 207
Autonomic nervous system, 112–113, 115

Autonomic respiratory center, 25–26, 25f
Axis alignment, 173, 174f, 205, 205f

B

Backward, upward, rightward pressure (BURP), 208
Bag-valve-mask ventilation
  equipment for, 104f
  in obese patient, 270
  pearls for, 104–105
  positioning for, 104f, 204f
  reservoir bag size for, 106
  tidal volumes for, 105
Barrel chest, 144, 146f
Base excess (B.E.), 42
Beclomethasone, 124
Benzodiazepines, 178–179
Beta agonists
  for asthma, 123
  for COPD, 125
  mechanisms of action of, 116–117
Bicarbonate/carbonic acid buffer system, 37
Bicarbonates
  in acidosis, 40, 42
  in alkalosis, 41, 42
  diffusion of, 24–25
  formation of, 24
Biot's respirations, 143t
Blood
  oxygenation of, 22–23, 53–55, 83. See also Hemoglobin; Pulse oximetry
  pH, 35
Boyle's law, 17
Bradycardia, with succinylcholine, 185
Bradypnea, 143t
Breath sounds, 143t, 236
Breathing (pulmonary ventilation), 16–18, 17f, 19f
Bronchi, 9–11, 10f
Bronchial artery, 16
Bronchioles, 11
Bronchiolitis, 242–243
Broncho-pulmonary dysplasia (BPD), 243–244
Bronchoconstriction, 112
Bronchospasm, 79, 82f

Buffer response
   renal (metabolic), 38
   respiratory, 37–38, 37*f*
Burn injuries, 263–265
BURP (backward, upward, rightward pressure), 208

C

Calcium antagonist overdose, 287
Capnography. *See also* End-tidal carbon dioxide (ETCO$_2$)
   in asthma/COPD exacerbations, 79
   in cardiopulmonary resuscitation, 78–79
   definition of, 72
   for early warning of shock, 80
   via endotracheal tube, 77
   for intubation verification, 77–78
   principles of, 72, 74, 80–81, 80–82*f*
   versus pulse oximetry, 77
   during transport of ventilated patients, 78
   uses of, 72–73, 77–80
   in ventilator weaning, 79–80
Carbaminohemoglobin, 98
Carbon dioxide
   in alveolar air, 96*t*
   in atmospheric air, 96*t*
   diffusion of, 21, 21*f*, 24–25, 73–74
   excretion of, 74
   production of, 73
   relationship with hydrogen ions and bicarbonate ions, 24
   transport of, 23, 74, 98–99
Carbon monoxide poisoning
   blood gas values in, 64*t*
   management of, 264–265
   pathophysiology of, 264
   pulmonary edema in, 288
   skin color in, 65
Carboxyhemoglobin, pulse oximetry accuracy and, 84–85
Cardiac arrest
   capnography during, 78–79
   oxygen use following, 73
   in pediatric patients, 234
Cardiopulmonary resuscitation
   capnography during, 78, 82*f*

   drug delivery during, 35–36
   oxygen use with, 73
Cartilage
   bronchial, 11
   thyroid, 7
   tracheal, 8
Catecholamines, 113
Central nervous system, 112, 115*f*
Central neurogenic hyperventilation, 143*t*
Cerebral perfusion pressure (CPP), 260
Chest injury, intubation in, 213
Chest x-ray, in pneumonia, 153
Cheyne-Stoke respirations, 143*t*
Children. *See* Pediatric patients
Chin lift, 202
Chloride shift, 99
Chronic bronchitis, 144–145, 144*t*. *See also* Chronic obstructive pulmonary disease (COPD)
Chronic obstructive pulmonary disease (COPD)
   exacerbation, capnography during, 79, 82
   physiology of, 124, 144–145
   signs and symptoms of, 125, 144–146, 145*t*
   treatment of, 125, 289
Clonidine, 114
Codeine, 118
Combitube. *See* Esophageal-tracheal double-lumen airway (Combitube)
Compensation, 46–47
Compliance, lung, 18
Congenital heart disorders, 67
Congenital subglottic stenosis, 248–249
Continuous positive airway pressure (CPAP)
   contraindications to, 290
   indications for, 289
   nasal, in premature infants, 15
   principles of, 288–289
COPD. *See* Chronic obstructive pulmonary disease (COPD)
Cor pulmonale, 158
Corticosteroids
   for asthma, 123–124
   for COPD, 125
   with etomidate, in rapid sequence intubation, 176

Cough, 117–120. *See also* Asthma
CPAP. *See* Continuous positive airway pressure (CPAP)
Crackles, 143*t*, 236
Cricoid pressure, 173–174
Cricothyroidotomy
  contraindications to, 275
  indications for, 274–275
  landmarks for, 274*f*
  needle, 278–279
  procedure for, 275, 276–278*f*
Cromolyn, 122
Croup (parainfluenza virus), 237
Croup (cool mist) tent, 100
Crouzon syndrome, 246, 247*f*
Cyanide poisoning, 65
Cyanosis, 64–65, 157

D

Dalton's law, 20–21, 95
Dead space ventilation, 76
Decongestants, 120
Demulcents, 118–119
Dexamethasone, 127, 176
Dextromethorphan, 118
Diaphragm, in respiration, 17
Diastolic dysfunction, 147
Difficult endotracheal intubation
  approach to, 212
  BURP maneuver for, 208
  causes of, 212–214, 212*t*, 213*f*
  elastic bougie for, 209–210, 209*f*
  esophageal-tracheal double-lumen
    airway for. *See* Esophageal-tracheal
    double-lumen airway (Combitube)
  fiberoptic bronchoscope for, 210
  larger blade for, 208
  laryngeal mask airway for. *See* Laryngeal
    mask airway (LMA)
  laryngeal tube for. *See* Laryngeal tube (LT)
  lighted stylet for, 208
  retrograde guide wire for, 212
Diffusion
  of carbon dioxide, 21, 21*f*, 24–25,
    73–74
  factors affecting, 96

  impaired, 68
  of oxygen, 20, 21*f*, 96
Diphenhydramine, 128–129
Diuretics, for cardiogenic pulmonary edema,
  148
Dobutamine, 117
Dopamine, 113, 115
Down's syndrome (trisomy 21), 247, 248*f*
Dyshemoglobinemias, 84–85
Dyspnea, 143, 157

E

Elastic bougie, 209–210, 209*f*
Elderly patients, airway management in,
  272–273
Emphysema, 145–146, 145*t*. *See also*
    Chronic obstructive pulmonary disease
    (COPD)
End-tidal carbon dioxide ($ETCO_2$). *See also*
    Capnography
  definition of, 72, 74
  $PaCO_2$ and, 76, 79
Endotracheal intubation. *See also* Rapid
    sequence intubation (RSI)
  assessment in, 198–200
  capnography for confirmation of, 77–78, 82*f*
  in chest injury, 213
  complications of, 195, 196–197, 197*t*
  difficult. *See* Difficult endotracheal intubation
  equipment and materials for, 198, 199–200*f*
  examination in, 200–201
  with full stomach, 212
  in head and neck injury. *See* Head injured
    patients
  history in, 201
  indications for, 195
  in intoxicated patients, 213
  in obese patients. *See* Obese patients
  objective criteria for, 196
  in pediatric patients. *See* Pediatric patients,
    intubation in
  in pregnant patient. *See* Pregnant patients
  procedure, 204–208, 204*f*, 205*f*, 206*f*, 207*f*
  subjective criteria for, 195
  suctioning for, 203
Endotracheal tubes, 199*f*

Epiglottis, 7
Epiglottitis, 237–239
Epinephrine
 for anaphylactic reaction, 130
 as neurotransmitter, 113
 pharmacology of, 129–130
 for wheezing in pediatric patients, 243
Esophageal intubation, 196, 197t
Esophageal-tracheal double-lumen airway
  (Combitube)
 advantages of, 211, 225
 characteristics of, 211f, 226–227f
 indications for, 211–212, 224–225
Etomidate, in rapid sequence intubation
 clinical actions of, 173t, 176
 corticosteroid use with, 176
 dosing of, 173, 173t, 176
 frequency of use of, 175
 as sole agent, 189–190
 in trauma patient, 257
Eupnea, 143t
Expectorants, 119
Expiration (exhalation), 18, 19f
Expiratory reserve volume (ERV), 19
External (pulmonary) respiration, 21–22, 21f

F

Facilitated intubation, 189
Fasciculations, with succinylcholine, 186–187
Fentanyl, in rapid sequence intubation,
  171–172, 173t, 257
Fiberoptic intubation, 210
"Fight-or-flight" response, 112
Fluticasone, 124
Foreign body aspiration (FBA), 239–240f,
  239–241
Functional residual capacity, 144, 269, 289
Furosemide, for cardiogenic pulmonary edema,
  148

G

Geriatric patients, airway management in,
  272–273
Goldenhar syndrome, 245
Guaifenesin, 119

H

Head injured patients
 critical care paramedicine in, 260–261
 endotracheal intubation in, 213–214
 ICP monitoring in, 260
 initial resuscitation in, 262
 prehospital treatment in, 261–262
 primary versus secondary, 259–260
 pulmonary edema in, 150
Head tilt, 201–202
Heart failure, 288
Hemoglobin
 carbon dioxide transport by, 98–99
 oxygen affinity for, 22–23, 52–53, 54f,
   97–98, 97f
 oxygen carrying capacity of, 97
 structure of, 52–53, 52f
Hemoglobin-buffer system, 37
Hering-Breuer reflex, 26
High altitude pulmonary edema, 149, 287–288
Hilus, lung, 13
Histotoxic hypoxia, 64t, 65
Hyaline cartilage, 8, 9f
Hydrocortisone, 176
Hyperemia, pulse oximetry in, 88–89
Hyperkalemia, with succinylcholine,
  184–185
Hyperpnea, 143t
Hyperventilation
 capnography during, 78, 79, 82f
 central neurogenic, 143t
 characteristics of, 143t
 for head injury, 261
 physiology of, 27, 27f
Hypoventilation
 blood gas values in, 66
 capnography during, 78, 82f
 causes of, 66
 during oxygen therapy, 106
 physiology of, 27, 28f
 pulse oximetry accuracy in, 89
Hypoxemia, 64t, 66–69
Hypoxia
 blood gas values in, 64t
 causes of, 63–64
 definition of, 62

Hypoxia (*Cont.*):
  pathophysiology of, 62–63
  pulse oximeter response to, 87
  signs and symptoms of, 65–66
Hypoxic drive, 110–111, 145
Hypoxic hypoxia, 64

I

Increased intraocular pressure, with
    succinylcholine, 186
Infants. *See* Pediatric patients
Inflation reflex, 26
Inhalation injury, 263–264
Inspiration (inhalation), 17–18, 17f
Inspiratory reserve volume (IRV), 19
Inspired oxygen (PIO₂), low, 66
Internal (tissue) respiration, 21f, 22
Intoxicated patients, intubation in, 213
Intracranial pressure (ICP)
    in head injury, 260
    monitoring, 260
    with succinylcholine, 186
Ipratropium bromide
    for asthma, 123
    for COPD, 125
    mechanisms of action of, 111, 130
    pharmacology of, 130–131
Isoetharine, pharmacology of, 131
Isoproterenol, 116–117

J

Jaw thrust, 202

K

Ketamine, in rapid sequence intubation, 173t,
    175, 177–178
Kussmaul's respirations, 143t

L

Laryngeal mask airway (LMA)
    advantages of, 220
    characteristics of, 210, 210f, 220f
    contraindications to, 222–223
    history of, 219
    indications for, 221–222
    insertion of, 223–224, 224t, 225f
    sizing of, 223t
    types of, 221
Laryngeal tube (LT)
    characteristics of, 227, 228f
    contraindications to, 228
    insertion of, 228, 229–231f
    sizing of, 230f
Laryngeal tube suction (LTS), 229
Laryngopharynx, 6
Laryngoscope blades, 200f, 206f, 208
Laryngospasm, 7, 197, 197t
Larynx
    anatomy and physiology, 6–8, 7f
    in pediatric patients, 235
Leukotriene pathway inhibitors, 124
Lidocaine, in rapid sequence intubation,
    171–172, 189, 259
LOAD mnemonic, for rapid sequence
    intubation pretreatment drugs,
    172, 172f
Lobules, 13
Loop diuretics, for cardiogenic pulmonary
    edema, 148
Lung sounds, 143t, 236
Lungs
    anatomy and physiology, 11–14
    blood supply, 16
    buffer response, 37–38, 37f
    compliance, 18
    pharmacology of drugs affecting, 111–112,
        126–136
    in pulmonary ventilation, 16–18, 17f, 19f
    volume and capacity, 19–20

M

Macintosh blade insertion, 206f
Magnesium sulfate, 131–133
Mainstream analysis, 77
Malignant hyperthermia, 184
Mallampati score, 212, 213f
Mannitol, 261

Mechanical ventilation, capnography during, 78
Medullary rhythmicity center, 25–26
Metabolic acidosis
    ABG values in, 44–45
    causes of, 40
    compensated, 51–52
    definition of, 40
    signs and symptoms of, 40
    treatment of, 41
Metabolic alkalosis
    ABG values in, 44
    causes of, 41
    compensated, 48–49
    definition of, 41
    signs and symptoms of, 41
    treatment of, 41
Metaproterenol
    for asthma, 123
    pharmacology of, 133–134
Methemoglobinemia, pulse oximetry accuracy in, 84–85
Methylprednisolone, 134–135
Methylxanthines, 122
Midazolam
    in head injury, 260
    in rapid sequence intubation, 173t, 178–179, 257
Minute volume of respiration (MVR), 19
Mitral stenosis, 147
Morphine
    for cardiogenic pulmonary edema, 148
    in head injury, 260
Motion artifacts, in pulse oximetry, 88–89
Mucolytics, 119
Mucous membrane, of larynx, 8
Muscarinic antagonists, 112, 123

N

Nail polish, pulse oximetry accuracy and, 87
Narcotic overdose, 149, 286–287
Nasal continuous positive airway pressure (NCPAP), in premature infants, 15
Nasal prongs (cannula), 99, 100, 100f, 101t
Nasopharyngeal airway, 202
Nasopharynx, 6

Near-drowning, 288
Neck injury, intubation in, 213–214
Nedocromil, 122
Needle cricothyroidotomy, 278–279
Neuromuscular blockers, in rapid sequence intubation
    critical factors in use of, 181–182
    depolarizing. See Succinylcholine
    mechanisms of action of, 181
    non-depolarizing, 187–189
    pharmacology of, 182
    in trauma patients, 258
Neuromuscular junction, 179–180
Neurotransmitters
    acetylcholine, 180–181
    of autonomic nervous system, 113
Nitrogen
    in alveolar air, 96t
    in atmospheric air, 53, 96t
Nitroprusside, for cardiogenic pulmonary edema, 148
Non-depolarizing neuromuscular blocking agents, in rapid sequence intubation, 187–189
Non-rebreather (reservoir) mask, 100–101, 101f, 101t
Norepinephrine, 113, 115
Nose, 4–6

O

Obese patients
    airway effects of pregnancy in, 268
    bag-valve-mask ventilation in, 270
    positioning for intubation in, 270–271, 271f
    posttracheal intubation management in, 271–272
    pulmonary physiology in, 269
Organophosphate poisoning, 114
Oropharyngeal airway, 202
Oropharynx, 6
Orthopnea, 143t
Osteopetrosis, 247–248
Oxygen
    affinity for hemoglobin, 22–23, 52–53, 54f, 97, 97f

Oxygen (*Cont.*):
  in alveolar air, 96*t*
  in atmospheric air, 94, 95, 96*t*
  diffusion of, 20, 22, 96
  measurement of, in blood, 53–55, 55*f*.
    See also Pulse oximetry
  nitrogen and, 53
  partial pressure of, 54, 94–96, 95*f*
  pharmacology of, 135
Oxygen delivery systems
  aerosol mask, 102, 103*f*
  bag-valve-mask, 103–106, 104*f*
  conserving devices, 99
  enclosure devices, 99–100
  hazards and complications of, 106
  high-flow devices, 99
  low-flow devices, 99
  nasal prongs, 99, 100, 100*f*, 101*t*
  non-rebreather (reservoir) mask, 100–101,
    101*f*, 102*t*
  purpose of, 99
  tank duration calculation, 106–107
  Venturi masks, 101, 102*f*, 103*t*
Oxygen-hemoglobin (oxyhemoglobin)
  dissociation curve, 23, 54, 55*f*, 97, 97*f*
Oxygen powered ventilators, 103–104, 105*f*
Oxygen saturation (SaO_2), 83. *See also* Pulse
  oximetry
Oxygenation, 74–75

P

$PaCO_2$
  in acidosis, 38, 42
  in alkalosis, 39, 42
  $ETCO_2$ and, 72, 76, 79
  versus $PeTCO_2$, 77
Pancuronium, 251
PaO_2, 52
Parainfluenza virus (croup), 237
Parasympathetic nervous system, 112–113
Partial pressures, 20, 94–96, 95*f*, 96*t*
Pediatric patients
  airway characteristics in, 235–236, 235*f*
  bacterial upper airway infection in,
    237–239

  broncho-pulmonary dysplasia in, 243–244
  conditions associated with difficult airway in,
    244–249, 245*f*, 246*f*, 247*f*
  croup in, 237
  foreign body aspiration in, 239–240*f*,
    239–241
  intubation in
    confirmation of, 252–253, 252*f*
    equipment for, 250–251
    indications for, 250
    laryngoscopy for, 249–250, 249*f*
    neuromuscular blockade for, 182, 185, 251
    preoxygenation for, 171
    pretreatment/sedative drugs for, 172, 176
    risks of, 250
    securing of tube following, 253–254,
      254–255*f*
    technique for, 251–252
Peripheral nervous system, 115*f*, 116*f*
$PeTCO_2$, versus $PaCO_2$, 77
pH
  in acidosis, 38, 40, 42
  in alkalosis, 39, 41, 42
  in arterial blood gas interpretation.
    See Arterial blood gas (ABG)
  of blood, 35
  in compensated acid-base disorders, 47
  scale, 35, 36*f*, 38*f*
Pharyngeal wall, 6
Pharynx, 6
Phenylephrine, 114, 120
Phosphate-buffer system, 37
Physiologic shunt, 67
Physiological buffer systems, 36–37
Pierre Robin syndrome, 244, 245*f*
PIO_2, 66
Pirbuterol, 123
Pleura, 11–12
Pleural cavity, 11
Pleural fluid, 11–12
Pleural friction rub, 143*t*
Pneumonia
  aspiration, 151
  bacterial versus viral, 154–155
  community acquired, 150–151
  complications of, 152

diagnosis of, 153
hospital acquired, 151
pathophysiology of, 152
signs and symptoms of, 154–155
treatment of, 155
ventilator-associated, 151
Pneumotaxic area, 26
Positive end-expiratory pressure (PEEP), 288
Potassium iodide, 119
Pralidoxime, 114
Preeclampsia, 267–268
Pregnant patients
airway assessment in, 267
airway management in, 171, 266–267
morbid obesity in, airway effects of, 268
preeclampsia in, airway effects of,
267–268
Premature infants
respiratory distress syndrome in, 14–15
Preoxygenation, for rapid sequence intubation,
171
Pretreatment drugs, in rapid sequence
intubation, 171–172, 172*f*
Primary bronchi, 9–10
Prolonged neuromuscular blockade,
with succinylcholine, 185–186
Propofol
in head injury, 260
in rapid sequence intubation, 173*t*, 179
Protein-buffer system, 37
Pseudoephedrine, 120
Pulmonary air volumes and capacities,
19–20
Pulmonary artery, 16
Pulmonary edema
cardiogenic, 147–149
CPAP for, 289. *See also* Continuous positive
airway pressure (CPAP)
neurogenic, 150
non-cardiogenic, 149–150, 286–288
pathophysiology of, 284–286
Pulmonary embolism, 150
Pulmonary hypertension, 158
Pulmonary vein, 16
Pulmonary ventilation (breathing), 16–18,
17*f,* 19*f*

Pulse oximetry
accuracy at different saturation levels,
84–85
versus capnography, 88
conditions affecting accuracy and precision of,
85–89
delay in detection of hypoxia with, 87
in dyshemoglobinemias, 84–85
in hyperemia, 88–89
in hypoventilation, 89
in hypoxia, 87
motion artifacts in, 88
principles of, 83

R

Racemic epinephrine, 135–135, 237
Rapid sequence induction, 166–167
Rapid sequence intubation (RSI). *See also*
Endotracheal intubation
advantages of, 169–170
axis alignment in, 173, 174*f*
contraindications to, 169
disadvantages of, 170
indications for, 168–169
modification of, 189
neuromuscular blockade for.
See Neuromuscular blockers
pretreatment drugs for, 171–172, 172*t*
procedure for, 170–175
versus rapid sequence induction,
166–167
sedative/induction agents for, 173*t*,
175–179, 257
in trauma patient, 256–259
Raynaud's disease, 86
Re-expansion pulmonary edema, 149
Renal artery stenosis, 147
Renal (metabolic) buffer response, 38
Residual volume (RV), 20
Respiration
control of, 25–27, 25*f*
dysfunction of, 27, 27*f,* 28*f. See also*
Respiratory failure
external, 21–22, 21*f*
internal, 21*f,* 22

Respiration (*Cont.*):
  pulmonary ventilation, 16–18
  purpose of, 16
Respiratory acidosis
  ABG values in, 43
  causes of, 38–39
  compensated, 46–48, 49–50
  definition of, 38, 38*f*
  signs and symptoms of, 39
  treatment of, 39
Respiratory alkalosis
  ABG values in, 45–46
  causes of, 39–40
  definition of, 39–40
  signs and symptoms of, 40
Respiratory buffer response, 37–38, 37*f*
Respiratory distress syndrome (RDS),
      in premature infants, 14–15
Respiratory failure
  acute versus chronic, 156
  causes of, 158–160
  classification of, 155–156
  definition of, 155
  diagnosis of, 154–157
  hypercapnic, 155–156
  hypoxemic, 155, 156
  pathophysiology of, 156
  in pediatric patients, 234
  signs and symptoms of, 157–158, 234
  treatment of, 160–161
Respiratory patterns, 142*t*–143*t*
Respiratory pharmacology. *See also*
      specific drugs
  for asthma, 122–124
  for COPD, 126
  for cough, 117–120
  emergency, 126–136
Respiratory syncytial virus (RSV), 242
Respiratory system
  conducting system, 4
  functions, 2–3
  lower, 3, 6–14, 7*f*, 9*f*, 10*f*, 12*f*
  in pediatric patients, 235–236, 235*f*
  upper, 3, 4–6, 5*f*
Return of spontaneous circulation (ROSC),
      capnography during, 79, 82*f*
Rhonchi, 143*t*

Right-to-left shunt, 67
Rocuronium, in rapid sequence intubation,
      188, 258
RSI. *See* Rapid sequence intubation (RSI)

S

Salicylate intoxication, 287
Salmeterol, 123
Sellick's maneuver, 173–174
Shock, capnography for early detection of, 80
Shunt perfusion, 76–77
Side-stream analysis, 77
"Sniffing" position, 205, 205*f*
Snoring, 236
SOAPME mnemonic, for intubation, 170
Stagnant hypoxia, 64*t*, 65
Status asthmaticus, 243
Stridor, 236
Subglottic stenosis, 248–249
Succinylcholine
  advantages of, 183
  bradycardia with, 185
  contraindications to, 184, 258
  dosing of, 183, 251, 258
  fasciculations and, 186–187
  hyperkalemia and, 184–185
  increased intracranial pressure and, 186
  increased intraocular pressure and, 186
  malignant hyperthermia and, 184
  mechanisms of action of, 182–183
  in pediatric patients, 185, 251
  prolonged blockade with, 185–186
  in trauma patient, 258
  trismus and, 186
Suction, airway, 203
Supraglottic airway device (SAD),
      218–219. *See also* Esophageal-tracheal
      double-lumen airway (Combitube);
      Laryngeal mask airway (LMA);
      Laryngeal tube (LT)
Surfactant, 13
Surfactant deficiency, 14–15
Swallowing, 7
Sympathetic nervous system, 112
Sympathomimetic agents, for asthma, 123
Systolic dysfunction, 147

T

Tachypnea, 142*t*
Terbutaline, 123, 136
Theophylline, 125, 127
Thiopental, in rapid sequence intubation, 173*t*, 176–177, 257
Thyroid cartilage, 7
Tidal volume (TV)
    on bag-valve-mask ventilation, 105
    definition of, 19
Trachea
    abnormalities of, 248
    anatomy and physiology, 8–9, 9*f*
    in pediatric patients, 235, 235*f*
Trauma patients, airway management in, 256–259
Treacher Collins syndrome, 245, 246*f*
Triamcinolone, 124
Trismus, with succinylcholine, 186
Trisomy 21 (Down's syndrome), 247, 248*f*
Type I alveolar cells, 13, 14*f*
Type II alveolar cells, 13, 14*f*

U

Upper airway infection, in pediatric patients, 237–239

V

Vagal stimulation, 197
Vapor pressure, 95–96
Vecuronium, 258
Ventilation, 75, 75*f*
Ventilation-perfusion dissimilarity, 67–68
Ventilation-perfusion relationship, 76–77
Ventilator-associated pneumonia, 151
Ventilator weaning, capnography during, 79–80
Venturi masks, 101, 102*f*, 103*t*
Vital capacity, 20
Vocal cord visualization, 206*f*
Voice production, 8

W

Water vapor
    in alveolar air, 96, 96*t*
    in atmospheric air, 95–96, 96*t*
Waveforms, in capnography, 80–81, 80*f*, 81*f*, 82*f*
Wheezing, 143*t*, 236, 243

Z

Zafirlukast, 124
Zileuton, 124